Work in Progress

~~Workin paoress~~

Work in Progress

Second Edition

Sarah E. Turner
Sue Dinitz
Kate Hoffman

The Writing Program
University of Vermont

Pearson Custom Publishing

Grateful acknowledgment is made to the following source for permission to reprint material copyrighted or controlled by it: "Sound of Silence," lyrics by Paul Simon and Art Garfunkel, 1966. Copyright © 1966 by Simon and Garfunkel/SONY/Columbia.

Printed in the United States of America.

10 9 8 7 6 5 4 3 2 1

Please visit our web site at www.pearsoncustom.com

ISBN 0–536–63372-x

BA 993197

Pearson Custom Publishing

PEARSON CUSTOM PUBLISHING
75 Arlington Street, Suite 300, Boston, MA 02116
A Pearson Education Company

Table of Contents

Personal Writing

Interpreting Texts

Research-Based Writing

Portfolio Narratives

Acknowledgments

Many people were involved in this project and in the creation of this text; we would like to thank the Center For Teaching and Learning for their generous support of this project. As well, Toby Fulwiler and the Writing Across the Curriculum program added both financial and moral support. Without the technical prowess of our editorial assistant Kate Hoffman, this book would not have come into being. In addition, we are indebted to the instructors of English 1 who not only gave us their student papers, but also gave most generously of their time: Steve Candiotti, Matthew Chipman, Megan Daum, Elizabeth Eschholz, Cristina Flores, Paul Hochanadel, Kate Hoffman, Bess Huddle, Kris Lamoreau, Robin Rapoport. But, most importantly, we would like to thank the students who were willing to allow us to use their voices and their work.

Introduction

This book represents our realization as instructors of English 1 that students would benefit from a common set of readings to facilitate conversation among the different sections and experiences of English 1 classrooms. Based on our classroom experience and on the input from our own students, we feel strongly that these readings should be essays written by students in English 1 rather than a collection of previously published essays. Such essays contribute to an understanding of the writing process; as you read these essays, you will see writers at work in various stages of this process. We hope this book encourages you to join them in the community of writers that make up not only your English 1 classroom but also your experience here at UVM.

Please keep in mind that our purpose was **not** to provide models showing what your own papers should look like. Rather, we hope these papers show you possibilities: possibilities for topics, for language, for shapes and forms, for beginnings and endings, for what can happen in the drafting, revising and editing processes, title construction, for almost any aspect of writing. Because we were looking for "works in progress," we did not ask the writers to further revise and edit their pieces; indeed, many of the texts aren't the writer's "final" draft. Instead, these papers illustrate a variety of approaches, voices, styles and purposes that you may identify with and perhaps draw upon as you work to develop your own writing style.

The book is organized into four sections, one for each of the three types of assignments commonly given in English 1: a paper based on personal experience, a paper interpreting a text, and a paper based on library and field research, as well as portfolio narratives. For each type of paper, we include at least one entire sequence of drafts, so you can see how the writer experimented with possibilities and how the paper evolved.

How did we choose which papers to include? We invited recent English 1 instructors to submit for consideration papers written by their students. Then a group of these instructors met with us in a day-long workshop, during which we selected a group of papers for each assignment that we thought would lend themselves to classroom activities. We change this book each year to include papers from current classes, so we hope you will consider submitting some of your own writing for next year's book and students.

Personal Writing

Timeline

Jennifer Collier

- Riding on the back of the bike with Ritchie and Ronny
- Walking to Shayla's
- Trying to leave Kara's
- The octagonal window in the closet
- The big yellow room
- Homer Bomer
- Moving to Wilmington
- Buster Brown
- Totem Pole park
- Getting tonsils out
- Snowmobiling on Lake Ossipee
- Dad moves to NH
- Finding Spooky
- Food games with Kellie
- Car accident; Sean in cast
- Inca project
- Dad's house in Woburn
- Jenn, Rob, and Joe move in
- Disney World
- Friday's with Val, Kris, Diana, and Mel
- September 28th– Ian
- Trips with Ian, Mel, Dave, Jamie, and Rob
- Cruise to Bermuda
- Police at Ian's
- Cruise to Caribbean
- Getting into UVM
- Graduation
- Party
- Trip to Mexico
- Trip to Florida
- Moving into dorm room

Snapshot Draft

Jennifer Collier

Walking to Shayla's

On the tiny cul-de-sac known as Ruby Road was the large brown colonial that I called home for the first five years of my life. That road always seemed so long to me. In reality, there were only about ten houses on the street. When you're younger, however, everything seems larger, more overwhelming, and, many times, somewhat more exciting.

I was grateful that our house was the first one on the street. Always eager for the next thing to do, I was happy that I didn't have to spend any more time than absolutely necessary in our blue Subaru.

Once I was old enough, my mother would allow me to walk alone to Shayla's house. This kind of unbelievable freedom was almost too much to bear. The house, on the same side of the street as ours, the right side, was only two houses down from our own. However, the towering colonials, that looked strikingly like our own aside from color, which I passed while on the route of my journey seemed never ending.

My mother would walk me to the door. I would continue, but she would stay there by the door. Sure, Nicole was with me, but she was only seven. I thought there was nothing more frightening. As I walked down the driveway and took a left down the sidewalk, I would turn around to make sure that my mother was still watching through the window. She would smile and wave and I would feel a little better.

I would tiptoe past the red house on the left, which my young mind was convinced was inhabited by robbers. This was the part of the trip that required the most courage.

After what seemed like an hour, I would arrive to the familiarity of my friend's house. I would play until it was time to begin the adventure home.

Car Accident

It was time to begin the long ride home from New Hampshire back home to Mom's house. Dad had two cars, a Jetta and a Ford pickup truck. I much preferred the Jetta for the two and a half hour trip because it was much more room for the five of us to fit in. However, the boys, with their obsession with trucks and anything that goes vroom, insisted that we take the pickup home.

We pile into the pickup. Sean, Dad and me spanning the front seat and Nicole and Andy sit in the back seat of the cab. The upholstery was red and smelled of antifreeze and oil. The seats were cramped and uncomfortable. I mumbled to myself, but did not argue because I knew I never won when it came to my younger brothers.

On a long, winding New Hampshire back road, the truck moved along with the usual Sunday night traffic. Dad's window was open. I could smell the trees and the wind blew my long hair all around, tying it into knots.

I watched as a bee flew in through the window. After stinging Dad on the leg, the bee flew back out quietly. At the pinching feeling, Dad looked down at his leg. As he did so, the truck slowly drifted to the left.

All I remember is the seat belt pushing against my stomach with excruciating force. I couldn't hear or think anything as the truck spun around and around for what felt like hours. Finally the second impact with the parked van snapped reality back into my head. All I heard was someone yelling for me to get out of the truck, but the handle wouldn't work. Attempting to roll down the window, I saw the concerned faces of strangers running over to pull me out.

Having been the only one in the truck to leave through that side, I was alone as the kind strangers laid me down on the pavement, attempting to assess the possible damage. Dad came over, unable to walk straight from loss of blood. He apologized over and over, saying he just didn't see it coming. I was scared for him. I stared at the payphone, crying that all I wanted to do was call my mother.

I looked back at the once large pickup, totaled and leaking clear liquids onto the dry, hot pavement. I thought of what would have happened if we had taken the Jetta and I thanked my brothers for their love of that truck.

Graduation

As we all sat on the cold, hard chairs in perfect formation, not listening to a word of the hollow, practiced speech of the principal, I think we all had the same thought in our minds: I can't believe this is finally it. All the girls wore the same bright white shin-length gowns and matching caps. The boys looked much the same, in their ocean blue outfits.

The field was wet and the air smelled of newly cut grass. The air was warm and sky was clear. However, none of us were paying any attention to the weather or to really anything else for that matter.

Images of past graduation ceremonies went through my head. I remember feeling like that'll never be me. It always seemed like a world away. It seemed unreal that it was finally my time.

When I heard the principal call my name, it was as though it all moved in slow motion. I walked alone to the podium and smiled at my friends and classmates as I passed them, as if to silently say "We finally did it".

The blue leather case held what was possibly the most important document I had earned so far in my life. The blue of the sky that provided the backdrop as I watched my cap fly through the air had never looked so blue. After it was over, I hugged my friends and we walked together off the football field of a school to which I would not return.

Robbers' House

Draft 2

Jennifer Collier

It's never quite been determined when or how the unreasonable fear originated. All I knew in my young, four-year-old mind was that robbers lived in that house. The house was large and red, a fire engine red that I have come to hate. There was nothing particularly intimidating about this house; in fact, it looked much like my own, and every other house on Ruby Road for that matter. However, sometime in the three short years that I lived across from that fire engine red house, I convinced myself that there was nothing but danger and evil that resided in it.

Ruby Road was your typical suburban street in your typical suburban neighborhood. There were sidewalks on either side of the cracked, light gray pavement that was the street. There were dark oil stains on the curb in front of many of the houses. Because it was a cul-de-sac, there was never any traffic, so it was safe to park your car on the side of the road if the driveway was full. Virtually every house on the street contained a family with two parents and varying numbers of children. At two o'clock every day, the familiar screech of the school bus brakes made their cry, informing the parents that their children were home from school. During the weekends, the familiar smell of cookouts in the summer and fireplaces in the winter blanketed the air. It was the typical American neighborhood.

However, to me, there was a house that deviated from this idyllic picture. Looking back, I'm sure that it looked exactly the same as the other houses on the street. That lot must have appeared just as warm and inviting to the unknowing eye as my own familiar home. But I knew that there was in fact something much different, much more dangerous in that lot than anyone could imagine.

The fire engine red of that house meant danger. The trees were not light and green; their leaves did not blow softly in the wind, creating that rustling sound that I loved so much to listen to. There were trees like all the other houses, but they served the sole purpose of keeping the warm light of the sun from reaching dark, lifeless grass that made up the lawn.

Halloween was coming and I convinced myself that I would go up to that house and confront those robbers while they were so innocently giving their candy to the children that I played with everyday. They probably stole that candy.

That evening I ate dinner as fast as I could. Halloween was always my favorite time of the fall and the closer it got to six o'clock, the slower time went by. Finally, the time came to put on my glow-worm costume. The plastic smock and mask fit perfect and I was convinced that nobody would know it was me, which was a perfect feature when you will be confronting robbers about their evil deeds.

Six o'clock finally came and my father took both my sister Nicole and me by the hands. We started with the blue house across the street. We walked across the street for what seemed like miles because I knew what house came after this one. I walked as slowly as I could to the front steps of the house, trying to stall as long as possible. I finally reached the door after my sister yelled at me a few times for moving so slowly. She was so stupid. If she knew what was in store for us next, she'd be moving just as slowly as I was.

As we went back down those steps and walked towards the end of the driveway to where my father was standing, Nicole took out the candy we had just received out of her pillowcase and began to unwrap it. How could she possibly eat? Not only was my stomach tied in knots tighter than my sneaker laces, but it had also somehow migrated to my throat. My palms were sweating profusely and I was beginning to have difficulty breathing. My legs couldn't have been heavier if two sacks of sand were tied to my ankles. I heard my sister telling me to hurry up, but I just couldn't make myself walk any faster.

We made our way around the large evergreen that separated the blue house from that of the robbers. It came into view and I froze. The house seemed as though it had grown by about ten stories. It loomed above me and it's top windows made eyes that stared down at me, daring my to move further. The red of the paint suddenly looked black and even the leaves were dark, instead of the bright yellows and reds that decorated my yard. It seemed as though the whole house was laughing at me. An evil laugh that told me that if I came any closer, I would be the next victim.

I ran across the street without even looking both ways, as I had been told to do for as long as I could remember. Hit me; I don't care. Anything is better than falling victim to the robbers! My sister and father looked at me with confusion as I was now on the other side of the street trying to catch my breath. There stood lonely glow-worm doubled over and struggling for air.

I didn't confront the robbers that night. I didn't have the courage. But I convinced myself that if I had, my family would have been robbed, and I would have been to blame. Perhaps I should've been a super-hero instead of a glow-worm.

A Study of Children and Imagination

Draft 3

Jennifer Collier

Journal of Biochemistry *Volume XX, Issue XIV*

Imagination is the beginning of creation. You imagine what you desire, you will what you imagine, and at last you create what you will.
— George Bernard Shaw

Imagination is defined as the conscious mental process of evoking ideas or images of objects, events, relations, attributes, or processes never before experienced.[1] In the continuing series on the human brain and imagination, the *Journal of Biochemistry* has conducted a study of children, their imaginations, and the impression it has on their lives. This report will record the findings of that study.

No one uses imagination more in his or her everyday life than a child. They use their imaginations as a method of entertainment. Whether they are creating a new friend or an entire world to play in, children rely on their extensive ability to imagine each day. Studies have shown that two out of every five children have created an imaginary friend to play with.[2]

There are times when the images that children create are not always helpful tools for them. Using their powerful imaginations, children can find horror in everyday objects and danger in the innocent faces of strangers. It is difficult to assess exactly how these horrors begin or why exactly the targets cause the terror, and consequently, studies on these "imaginary horrors" are limited. The long-term effects that they have on the child have yet to be determined. However, it is easy to locate the immediate effects when speaking to the child.

Experts from the *Journal of Biochemistry* traveled to several small towns in northern Massachusetts. In these towns, they found several cases of this "imaginary horror" and interviewed the children experiencing it. This was done to avoid discrepancies that may have been caused by differing experiences.

The children were all the same age and came from similar socioeconomic backgrounds. Each had two siblings, two live-in parents, and had spent the entire four years of their lives free of any serious trauma or harm. Similarly, the towns and families in which each of the children grew up were very similar.

The researchers began first by interviewing the child and the parents together. They then interviewed each separately. For three hours each day, they observed the child playing with friends and interacting with family. After a second and final interview, the researchers concluded their study of that particular child and repeated the same steps with five other cases.

After all six children were interviewed and analyzed, the researchers compiled and evaluated all of the information gathered. The experiments and the research that followed yielded interesting new facts and raised questions that may result in the development of groundbreaking new theories in the field of child psychology.

For the purposes of this report, the researchers chose one particular case that raised the most questions. This was the case of a young girl from Dracut, Massachusetts named Jennifer Collier. There are no clues as to the origin of the child's fears. They seem to be based completely and solely on an imagined event in the child's mind.

The subject has lived in the same upper middle class neighborhood for her entire life. The area is very tranquil and quiet. There are many families with children close in age to our subject.

Her parents described the young subject as being extremely outgoing and energetic. "Jennifer has never had any problems with shyness. She has always been so talkative with strangers that it is even concerning sometimes. She also never seems to have any particular issue with fear, other than in this one case," explains Mrs. Collier, the subject's mother.

However, the child had quite an issue with fear when it came to one particular house in her neighborhood. In the following interview, the subject tells our researchers about the house across the street from her own.

Researchers from JBC: So, Jennifer, tell us about the house across the street from your home.

Jennifer Collier: Robbers live in that house.

JBC: How do you know that?

JC: I've seen them.
JBC: You've seen them robbing people?
JC: No.
JBC: How can you be sure that they are robbers?
JC: Because they are bad people.
JBC: Can you tell us what their house looks like?
JC: It is dark, dark red. It is very tall. There are huge windows that are always dark. The robbers never come outside because they are afraid that someone might see them. They only come out at night when they are going to rob someone.
JBC: Have you ever seen them come out at night?
JC: No, but that's the only time that they must come out because they don't come out in the daytime.
JBC: Have you ever told the robbers that what they are doing is wrong?
JC: I tried once, but it didn't work.
JBC: What happened?
JC: It was last Halloween and I was going trick-or-treating with my daddy and my sister. I decided to tell the robbers that night that I know what they are doing.
JBC: Is there any reason that you chose Halloween night?
JC: Because I was wearing a mask and they couldn't tell who I was.
JBC: You said that it didn't work. What happened?
JC: I got too scared. Nobody but me knows that they are robbers, so I had to go and tell them by myself. I was too afraid to do it.
JBC: Do you think that you will try again someday?
JC: Maybe. I just really hope that they will move away some day. Or that me and my mommy and daddy and sister will move away from the robbers before they rob us.

The child was observed to be very happy and outgoing when not talking about the house across the street. She chatted with strangers and played with the neighborhood children. No mental or personality disorders were revealed during the screening. She was friendly in her conversations with our researchers. However, somewhere in her imagination, she developed the idea that the innocent neighbors across the street from her home were a source of danger and evil. When she was questioned as to how she knew this, she was unable to give a concrete answer, but was confident that she was correct.

Many times, it has shown that such situations are harmless to the child. In fact, they are healthy. They show that the child is using his or her imagination. Some parents become concerned when a child creates such a disturbing situation in his or her head. They witness the terror that the child experiences and worry that it will continue to affect him or her later.

So far, our research has shown that this is not a serious problem. The child will grow out of the fear. He or she will learn over time that there is nothing, in fact, supporting the fear and will eventually let it go. It has actually been shown that such vivid images and thoughts are a healthy sign. It shows that the child is using the very important tool that all were born with and some ignore: the imagination.

The *Journal of Biochemistry* will continue the study of the human imagination with a piece on adults in the upcoming issue.

There is only one admirable form of imagination: the imagination that is so intense that it creates a new reality.

— Sean O'Faolain

[1] *Encarta Encyclopedia* 1998; Volume I

[2] *Journal of Medical Research*; Volume XXX, Issue XI

Snapshots

Krystopher Hettrick

Snapshot #1

When I was young, I perceived my little sister Leah as this innocent, little princess and thought that she was physically unable to harm anyone. I thought that since she was only four years old, she couldn't bother me, but that all changed the summer before I was supposed to start school. It was a beautiful July afternoon, and I was playing outside in the yard, while my dad mowed the lawn and did other chores around the house. The air smelled of freshly cut grass and there was a slight breeze. As I played around the yard, I realized that I hadn't played on the swing set in a long time. So, as I headed toward the back part of the yard towards the swings, I heard my mom yell to me. I turned around and saw my sister running towards me, as my mom said, "Watch Leah for me, I have to go to the store." I agreed and my mom left.

I don't particularly like to watch my sister, but I didn't have a choice. I figured a day with my sister would be a good bonding experience, boy was I wrong. My sister climbed up the slide and sat on the top. I then climbed the slide behind her and said I would give her a push to get her started. But, just then, she leaned backward and pushed me off the back of the slide. As I fell, I hit my arm on the tree directly behind the slide. I started to cry as soon as I hit the ground, I couldn't feel my right arm. My sister was laughing by then, I guess she thought it was funny. I got up and quickly followed the sound of the lawn mower toward my dad. He saw me crying and figured something was wrong, so after he realized my arm was probably broken, we got my sister and went to the emergency room. At the hospital I got a cast and a disability for six weeks. As I thought about what happened, I realized two things, my sister is the devil, and I won't be able to write for the first six weeks of my first year of school.

Snapshot #2

It was the moment that I have been waiting for all my life, the moment that I dreamt about many times. What would be so important? I am sixteen, have my driving learner's permit, and the day has come for the big test. Not only does a driver's license give you the right to drive, it also gives you freedom. It was November 4, 1998, and at 9:00 a.m. I had to be at the Connecticut Department of Motor Vehicles. I woke up at 7:00 a.m. because I was so excited that I couldn't sleep, and got ready in about fifteen minutes. I was so nervous I couldn't even eat breakfast, so I skipped it. My dad got ready and we started our journey along the "yellow brick road." My dad let me drive there, so I would get more practice. Finally, we got there, it was the weirdest place ever, there was a line out the door and all these high-tech machines.

After an hour of waiting, I took my eye test, and sat down in front of a computer screen to take my animated test, with pictures and everything. After doing great on the written part, it was time to show the inspector what I could do on the road. As I cruised down the street with two hands on the wheel, and the inspector barking out orders, everything seemed to go in slow motion. As all of my five senses were alert and working to show perfect textbook driving, I realized we were already back at the DMV. I parked the car, and the inspector said, "Congratulations, you passed your road test." I nearly kissed the inspector. I walked back into the building, told my dad, got my license, and drove home in triumph.

Snapshot #3

Besides the sporting events, in high school, the second thing that I remember very well is toilet papering. It was the night before the big cross town rival game between my school Maloney and the other school Platt. These two schools are mirror images of each other and every year on Thanksgiving they go head to head in one of the best football games of the year. My friends and I decided to toilet paper our school, because if we "vandalize" the other school, we could be arrested. We told everyone that we knew, and that night, when about one hundred people showed up with toilet paper we were surprised. I went to work on the trees, launching the rolls all the way to the top and watching them stream down, leaving a trail. After about two hours of work, the toilet papering crew, now dwindled, decided to retire for the night. As I left I looked back at the trees and wondered if they needed more toilet paper. This was one of the only times in my life that I was able to vandalize something and get away with it.

A Significant Fall

Draft 2

Krystopher Hettrick

When I was young, I perceived my little sister Leah as this innocent, little princess and thought that she was physically unable to harm anyone, especially me. I thought that since she was only four years old, and me being seven years old, she couldn't bother me. But, that all changed the summer before I was supposed to start my first year of elementary school.

It was a beautiful July afternoon, the birds were singing their amazing tunes while the sun was shining all over the great city of Meriden, Connecticut. The weather had been unusually awful for this time of year, so I was taking advantage of the great weather that we were having, and was playing outside in my yard. I was just running around the yard with every toy possible, trying to play everything all at once. "Too many toys, too little time." That day in particular, I was having a lot of trouble deciding whether I wanted to play with my G.I. Joe figures with kung-fu grip, or my He-man action figures. As I was running around the yard, my dad was mowing the lawn in super fast gear, as if he was a racecar driver, trying to win the Indianapolis 500. The air smelled of freshly cut grass and there was a slight breeze that made my parachuting G.I. Joe's float away.

As I was running to get my two parachuters when I caught a glimpse of the swing set and I realized that I hadn't played on it in a long time. That moment, I sent all my figurines flying and took off toward the fully accessorized swing set that my dad had built for my sister and I last year. I hit the bottom of the slide and went running up it like gravity had no effect on me. I was the King of the Slide, and nobody could take my crown away. I slide down the fire pole as if I was an actual firefighter going to a three-alarm fire. Not only was the swing set fun to play on, it was pretty good looking, it was silver and blue and it gleamed in the sunlit part of my yard. It almost looked like a futuristic castle, because to a seven year old, it looked massive. I started to play on the swings, they were so comfortable with their cushioned seats. I started off swinging slowly, then I began to pump my legs harder and harder, and

I started gaining momentum and speed. As the wind flew past my head, I got an adrenaline rush, and I realized that I was living on the edge.

My fun was soon ended when I heard my mom yell, "KRYS." I couldn't respond too well because I was swinging parallel to the top pole of the swing set. I spread my arms and legs out to try and slow myself down. My mom kept yelling, and I could tell that she was getting progressively mad as the tone in her voice went from calm to aggravated. Finally, I responded with an exhausted "Yes." Just then, my sister came running at me calling "Didter." She called me this because she couldn't say Krystopher and that was her version of my name. I thought it was really cute; I would always be able to tell when my sister was calling me because it was so high pitched and funny sounding that it stood out. I noticed that she had her hair in pigtails, and this matching pink t-shirt and shorts outfit on. My sister came right up to me and hugged me in the same moment without hesitating. While she embraced me, my mom yelled to me, "Watch Leah for me, I have to go to Shop Rite for groceries." Since I really couldn't say no, I was stuck with my sister for the next two hours or so, Great!

I didn't particularly like to watch my sister because its responsibility that at my age is like the whole world is being put on my shoulders. I don't know how to take care of a little child, I am one myself! Realizing at that moment that I didn't have a choice in the matter, I started to think how fun it would be to bond with my sister for a day. So, we started heading back towards the swing set. My sister loves the slide, so she didn't hesitate and headed straight for it. Leah climbed the slide and sat on the ledge waiting for me. I then climbed up the ladder of the slide right after her and told her that I would give her a push so that she may go faster. Just as I set up to give her a push, my little sister, the angel, leaned backward and nudged me off the slide. As I was falling, I hit my right arm on this big, thick maple tree that was two feet behind the slide. I didn't even hit the ground and I was already up running around the yard in tears. I was just running, in circles, in lines, I didn't know what to do. I couldn't move my arm, and it bruised almost immediately. My sister obviously thought that it was funny and was laughing by now.

I came to my senses and realized that I needed to tell my dad what happened and have him help me out. I sprinted across that yard, following the sound of the blade of the lawnmower. I caught up to him in the front yard and he knew as soon as he saw my tear-covered face that something was wrong. My dad is a police officer, so I don't know why he decided that he should start trying to figure out what was wrong with my arm. He started to poke and squeeze at it, boy did that hurt. Either way, my dad is a very smart man, and he sensed that my arm could possible be broken. He ran inside to get the keys to the car, rounded up the culprit who broke my arm, and we all packed into the car. Destination-Hospital.

I think of myself as a considerably tough kid, so as I was walking into the emergency room, with my tears faded away, I thought I could handle this. But, as I got into the waiting room and viewed all these kids there crying, I couldn't hold back my tears and started to ball. We checked in at the nurses' desk and then went to sit down. I looked around the waiting room and saw these pictures that I couldn't make heads or tails of. I was doing anything to keep my mind off my arm. My dad asked me to get a magazine for us, so I ventured over to the big wooden rack on the wall. I looked at the selection and decided to get the July Sports Illustrated. But, as I reached up to get it with my right arm, I realized that wouldn't work, so I used my left arm.

After about a half an hour of waiting and flipping through the pages of the magazine, the nurse yelled, "Hettrick." I pretty much jumped out of the chair and ran toward the open door. I just wanted the doctor to look at my arm and go home, besides, the smell of alcohol and astringent was making me feel light headed. First, I walked to this funny looking room with all these gigantic machines and laid down on a big table. Everybody then left the room and an object resembling a camera came down and took a picture of my outstretched arm. As this is happening, I am thinking what the heck could possible be going on. I have no clue and decide that the doctor is getting paid a great deal to do this, and he obviously knows what he is doing. After that was done, I asked my dad about the incident and he explained to me that it was an X-ray machine, and it was looking at my bone to tell whether or not it was broken.

Not soon after the X-ray room, I was walking to this other room that looked like a typical hospital room, with a bed and some heart monitoring machines. This was the part I liked least. The doctor came in and simple got straight to the point as he told my dad, "Krys' arm has a hairline fracture and he needs a cast." "Just great," I said. Not more than ten minutes after the orthopedic specialist came in I had a rock hard, white cast that would hinder my abilities as a kid. I was not very happy. I couldn't believe that I was unstoppable, and now I was temporarily handicapped for the next six weeks.

As I lay in my bed that night, just staring at the stupid white thing on my arm, I thought about what happened and how it could have been different. It was at that point in my life that I made a realization about my sister; she was a little, cute girl disguised as the Devil! I will have to keep an eye on her for the rest of my life if I want to avoid tragic accidents like this one.

THE RECORD-JOURNAL

July 21, 1989— Sibling rivalry taken to extremes

Krystopher Hettrick
Draft 3

Meriden, Connecticut— What has society come to? As the years go by, there seems to be an influx in the violence happening among little children under the age of ten. Yesterday's incident fits into that category. This incident has left one kid in the hospital and another not old enough to understand what she did.

At about three o'clock p.m. on Wednesday afternoon seven year old Krystopher Hettrick of 62 Ione Drive in Meriden was pushed off of the back of his swing set and suffered severe trauma to his right arm. The culprit who did this was no other than his four year old kid sister Leah. It started out to be a great day, no clouds in the sky and the birds were singing. Most of the neighborhood kids were playing outside in the sunshine; Krys was no exception. While his father mowed the lawn, he played outside with his toys.

At around 2:45 p.m. Kathy, Krys' mom, went to Shop Rite to buy some groceries and left Leah with Krys to play in the yard. As Kathy left, the two siblings headed toward the swing set to play. Leah climbed up the slide and Krys followed her. The both of them reached the top, and just as Krys was about to give his little sister a push down the slide, it happened. Leah struck Krys with her elbow and almost immediately he was airborne off the back of the slide. He then plummeted 6 feet to the ground, but not before maiming his arm on the big oak tree directly behind the slide. This event took place just moments after their mom left. Krys' father, Robert, quickly rushed his son to the emergency room where they diagnosed him with a fractured right arm. The doctor in charge of Krys quickly put a cast on his arm and sent him home to get some rest.

As for the juvenile delinquent who did this to him, she is serving no punishment because of lack of evidence. This incident just goes to show you how lenient our judicial system has become, where a kid can do anything she wants and get away with it. As for Leah, she is probably enjoying a tea party, while she still remains a threat to society. The swing set still remains a crime scene, littered with caution tape, and who knows if this incident will ever be solved and someone found responsible.

The Princess and the Slide

Draft 4

Krystopher Hettrick

My name is Leah, and my brother Krystopher and I used to do everything together, that is until one summer when a tragic accident occurred and caused him to become very cautious of me. I think that it was the summer when I was about to enter preschool, yeah, that's it.

It was one of those months during the summer; I am not sure which one though, because I am only four years old and I don't really know the names of the months yet. I had just gotten out of my little princess bed and decided to get dressed. My bed is very pretty; it is one of those wood beds, with the posts and a canopy on top. The sheets are Barbie design with all the different outfits that Barbie wears. I have my entire stuffed animal collection on the bed and it is cozy to sleep in. Like I was saying, my mom had just woken me up and I decided to get dressed and go outside to play. Mom set my clothes out for me, and I noticed that it was this little pink outfit with little flowers all over it. I loved it. I got dressed and waited for my mom to return to brush my hair. This is the most difficult part of my day. I hate getting my hair brushed. My hair is extremely curly and it hurts when my mom brushes it, because it pulls on my head.

Just then, my mom entered the room and I began to yell "No, No," when I saw her with a brush in her hand. I tried to run out of the room when my mom picked me up kicking and screaming and sat me in the chair. She held me in the chair with one hand and brushed my hair with the other hand. Finally I break loose from her grip and ran down the stairs as if I never even touched the stairs at all. I kind of just floated like an angel. I knew that my mom wouldn't follow me and try to brush my hair again, so I just waited for her to come down the stairs and make me breakfast. I was looking forward to my Lucky Charms cereal; I loved that cereal. I ate Lucky Charms everyday of the week, and nobody could make me change my mind.

As I sat down to my bowl of cereal, with my little kids spoon in hand, I noticed my brother playing outside with his

G.I. Joes. I was jealous that he was outside and I had to eat breakfast. I am a very sneaky kid, so I put my cereal back in the box and hurried down the stairs. But, as I did, my mom called out to me, "Leah, where are you going?" I told her that I was going to play with my brother, and she said, "Okay." I guess she didn't notice that I didn't eat my breakfast. As I opened the sliding door leading outside my mom followed me. I sprinted towards my brother who was now on our swing set, she said, "Krystopher, watch your sister for me while I go to Shop Rite to buy some groceries." I figured great, my brother is in charge of me, what does he know about taking care of little kids, he is only seven years old.

What a great day out, the birds were flying around the yard, this way and that, looking for worms and straw to make nests with. I loved to play in the sunlight, it made me feel all warm. I decided that my Barbies could wait for one day while I played outside with my brother; he always made everything fun because he was very creative. I ran straight toward the slide, I love the slide. I grabbed the ladder and took my time climbing up the ladder so that I didn't fall. As I climbed the ladder, my brother said, "I will give you a push so that you can go faster." I told him okay and waited for him to climb up the ladder. Just as he was about to give me a push a bee came flying near my head and I started to shoe it away. In the process of trying to get the bee away from me, I hit my brother with my elbow and knocked him off of the back of the slide.

When Krys hit the ground, he immediately got up and started running around the yard like a crazy man, I just figured that he was okay and went for a run. It was a pretty funny scene, so I started to laugh. Little did I know that it was serious. He ran up to the front of the yard and I lost sight of him. I just started sliding down the slide and playing on the swings. About five minutes later, my dad came running toward me, came over to me, picked me up and off we went running again towards the front yard. I was literally thrown into the backseat of the car as we sped away to an unknown place.

My dad, Krystopher and I arrived at this gigantic building and I didn't have a clue what the building was for. As we walked into the building I looked at the big blue letters and couldn't make heads or tails out of what it said, so I just followed and kept wondering where we could be. The inside of the building was like Barbie's dream house, it had all these nice colors, but it was mostly white with a lot of pretty things.

The halls were completely white and there were lights everywhere that made the building sparkle like a palace. Finally we reached this little room with a lot of seats and tables and my dad told me to sit down in one of the chairs and he would be right back. So, I picked a chair and sat down. As I looked around the room, I saw some people looking at magazines and just waiting for something.

I watched as my dad and brother went up to the front desk and talked to the lady behind the desk. After a short conversation, she handed my dad a whole bunch of papers. I was jealous because I wanted some paper to color on too. That was the moment when I knew why we were at this place. My dad told me that this was a hospital and we were here because there could be something wrong with Krystopher's arm that was caused by the fall. Just then I started to feel sorry for my big brother. I looked over at him and he was in pain, my poor big brother. My dad filled out the papers that were required by the hospital. Then Krys went over to the magazine rack and picked out a magazine for us to look at.

Less than a half an hour later the nurse came out into the waiting room and called "Hettrick." At that moment my dad and brother got up from their seats and started towards the door. My dad told me to wait here while the nurse that he asked would watch me. I had no choice but to sit there and look at all the decorations on the walls. While I was looking, I noticed something that I hadn't seen before, a television. I could hardly contain myself, that's what I do all day when I am not playing with my Barbies, I watch cartoons. The nurse got the remote and turned the cartoon network on for me while she watched me. I watched two or three shows before my father and brother walked back into the waiting room.

As they entered the waiting room, I noticed something different about my bigger brother, he had this funny white thing on his arm. It looked like it was part of his arm. When I pointed at it my brother said, "Shut up Leah, it is all your fault." My dad immediately told my brother to be quiet, we then left the hospital and went home in the car.

The rest of the night Krys stayed in his room and wouldn't talk to me or even acknowledge me, so it was back to playing Barbies for me. I thought to myself that it was such a long day, and I had been introduced to so many new places that at seven o'clock that evening I was tired and went to bed. I slept like a baby.

Portfolio Cover Letter

Ryan Corlis Trombly

Through this personal study it was clear to me that with each draft that I wrote my ability to convey my true feelings, and to open up as a writer greatly improved. From the beginning with the first drafts of snapshots I merely told of the significant events without sufficient detail and was unable to truly show the events to the reader. With the following draft I felt it important to focus on the details of one of these events, and felt successful in doing so. The detail of this draft improved the paper, but the true emotion and voice still was lacking. Rather than retell the story I decided to turn the paper into a journal format, with this I was able to reflect upon the story on a more personal level allowing for a greater sense of emotion and a stronger voice. Also writing this draft at such a personal level developed my ability to open up as a writer. The journal entry format was as far as I could go with that subject and felt that it was the best reflection of the event. The next draft involving the question, "Who Am I?" I decided to write a completely new piece as I felt it would be the only way to truly answer this question. I feel this draft was my best work, and was a great representation of where my development as a writer from step to step has led me. In the paper I incorporate nearly no aspects of prior papers feeling they did not define me and decided to do an overall self-evaluation of who I am. My thoughts were that the best way of doing this would be by examining my life at a glance, and then to take a closer look at the events of my life that determine who I am, and finally to examine who I have become. I definitely feel that this was my strongest paper and found it hard to revise, because it was exactly what I wanted to say. I felt that this paper would better fit my final draft, but decided to revise the paper by merely focusing on the poem portions of the prior paper. It was my opinion that poetry is written at a more free and open level and better conveys true feelings and descriptions. The last draft is more summarized than the prior draft without the opening paragraphs, with a shortened introduction, and with Emerson's quote presented at the beginning. In all honesty I feel that my fourth draft, *Sketches of Evaluation,* is the best representation of my development as a writer through this course.

In the end I feel that I accomplished what I wanted to more and more with each draft, and I feel that the final product of my portfolio is true and complete.

Timeline

Ryan Corlis Trombly

Birth 6/12/81
Senior trip to cancun, mex. (unreal)
First Phish concert Worcester Centrum, MA *12/29/95*
Caitrin
Road trips to Florida with family
75 gallon fish tank w/ African cichlids
Camp Mi Te Na 8th grade
State Champs CYO basketball NH-MVP

Severely injuring knee first day of school as sophomore in high school-changed lifestyle in first scrimmage of the year

job at Goodale's Bike & Ski trips to Burlington,vt with brother wrestling with friends-"to the death" David sunflower seeds

Playing basketball in Boston Garden before it got tore down Bedroom at home Dali

Chester Trpk. and Tower Hill Rd Central Pride
Grampy Corlis death

4 ideas from above write about in full detail
just write/ four separate due Wed 9/6

1. Caitrin
2. cancun, mex. trip
3. severe knee injury
4. fish tank

Events of Life

Snapshot Draft

Ryan Corlis Trombly

"Pittsburg, NH"

Every year, once a year, until my brother and I were both in high school we would go camping and fishing in Pittsburg, New Hampshire, the northernmost part of my home state. The week before we needed to return to school we would take the three-hour voyage northward to our favorite campground on Lake Francis to enjoy the wilderness and to really rough it. We would pack up the old musty tent, our sleeping bags, some shabby clothes, our fishing poles, and bare essentials and leave on the trip we looked forward to all through summer vacation.

Each year we would arrive and I would immediately choose which campsite it would be that we would stay at for the week, the only job assigned to me other than collecting kindling and wood so I took it seriously. I was the younger one so my father and brother took it easy on me, my brother was given such tasks as setting-up the tent, keeping the fire going, and even preparing dinner. It wouldn't take long for us to get established as the years went on, but nevertheless it was a hassle to do after sitting squished up against old smelly camping supplies in the a car during eighty degree weather for a little over three hours. The first day of the trip would always slip away into the still night sitting as we would sit beside the cozy campfire, drinking hot cocoa, and playing gin rummy. I don't believe that my life will ever encounter moments so peaceful as these.

For the remainder of the week we would be given beautiful daytime weather to fish the three Connecticut Lakes and to view the multitude of gigantic moose that mope around the area often strolling into the road or roaming beside it. The nights on the other hand would be a persistent majority of torrential downfalls where we would be awoken by buckets of water falling threw the roof of the tent that would be carelessly left uncovered by a tarp. My father would often laugh hardily as we all franticly ran around in the middle of the night, in the middle of a rainstorm, trying to salvage what dryness we could by now throwing the waterproof tarp into place.

The vacation was always a great experience for us three, it gave us time to bond with our father and to learn what he had to teach us, and it instilled in us the importance of nature and our environment. It brought us all closer to share these fond memories, from going to the dump to see black bears and having them almost attack the car to the time we collectively caught eighteen trout in a single day. It was our time together before we would grow up and go off on our own to live our own lives, it was the time for the three of us to share then, now, and always.

8th Grade Basketball State Champs

We had all played basketball together for the past six years on travel teams or school teams, the twelve of us had grown up in the small town of Hooksett, a majority of us even lived in the same neighborhood. Basketball was all we'd do, either on courts in our driveways, or at parks, and in the winter in gyms. Now we were all in eighth grade playing for the middle school team, the Hooksett Memorial Hawks, in the New Hampshire State championship game, which we had already won four years in a row. The significance of this game was not only the fact that we were competing for our school's fifth basketball consecutive championship or the fact that we were attempting to uphold five seasons of being not only champions but undefeated, but also it would be the last time that we all would play together on the same team. Due to the fact that we came from a small town that didn't have its own high school many of us would end up choosing different schools to attend.

All the emotions of a long hard season against the best competition in all of New Hampshire had culminated into one thirty-two minute game against an equally good team from Litchfield. We had played even the largest schools from cities such as Concord, Portsmouth, and Manchester and beat them all, but this Litchfield team had given us a scare earlier in the season as we only beat them by a couple points. Before the game we went threw the same ritual we had gone through since fifth grade, complete silence up until ten minutes before the game when we would erupt with claps and chants. This time had much more energy than ever as we ran out in a line onto the court to start the game. Never had I been more excited about getting something underway in my life.

The game started with great intensity as all of our pent up energy was released, I can't say that anyone of us had ever played better than we had that day. All twelve of us got a chance to shine as the game was quickly put away due to the talent of our team and individuals. By the second quarter of the game. we had a comfortable twelve point lead that kept rising as the game went on. I myself performed better than that day, as I ended the game with twenty-three points that led the team. With thoughts of leaving the security of our small town and close friends for different high schools in different towns behind us we peaked in our best performance ever, winning the game by twenty-eight points. For the last time on one team, "perhaps the most talented middle school basketball team of New Hampshire's athletic history," as the Manchester Union Leader wrote in its sports page, played its last game together.

I would have to say about eight of us went on to play varsity basketball at several different high schools in southern New Hampshire and had true impacts, but when we talk about those days now we all agree that we never played on another team better than our eighth grade championship team. Some of us have gone on to collegiate basketball, some have been injured, some just didn't want to play anymore, but all of us will remember the excitement and fun of playing basketball everyday of our childhoods, together, as teammates and friends.

Knee Injury

It was the day before the first day of school my sophomore year in high school, for the past two weeks I had strenuously worked to secure a position on the varsity soccer team during try-outs and it proved successful. The last two weeks had been filled with three-mile runs, practices, and team scrimmages, the fact that it all paid off and I made the varsity team left me ecstatic. My first time playing on the varsity team was a scrimmage against a lower division high school and was suppose to be a helpful warm-up before the real season began.

The scrimmage was on a cool overcast day in early September right before the brisk winds of autumn rolled in. The grass was damp from the dew left from the night before as the game started early in the morning. The coach told me to start the game so that I could get some more experience competing at the varsity level. Wanting to immediately impress the coach I put forth my fullest effort as I concentrated on not screwing up and hustling all over the field. Not even ten minutes into the game though my prior efforts and future goals were abruptly ended by the goalie of the opposing team.

The ball had traveled over several defenders heads and right to my feet as I streamed to the oppositions goal, quickly running I flew by the final defender and towards the goalie, who also sprinted forth from his position to stop my rush. Simultaneously as I planted my left leg and swung my right to kick the ball deep into the net the goalie lunged out at me and into my extended leg snapping it backwards and hyperextending it. I lied on the ground in intense pain as teammates, opponents, and coaches ran out to assist me aware of the severity due to just witnessing it.

I was rushed urgently to the Dr. Valais, an orthopedic surgeon who after examining my knee and the X-rays decided on setting my appointment for surgery for the following day. My knee had been hyperextended so badly that I tore two ligaments, snapped two tendons, torn cartilage, and broken my fibula. Needless to say my sports career was over, something that was quite hard for me to adjust to due to the large role that athletics played in my everyday life.

Each day after school I would need to attend rehabilitation sessions for two hours of excruciating pain. After months of this disheartening routine I was left with eighty-two percent strength in my left knee, and it wasn't going to get any better. Although this reality was difficult to deal with at first it was an adjustment I had to make in my life. Rather than playing competitive sports, I decided to participate in recreational activities and sports, such as CYO basketball, snowboarding, backpacking, fly-fishing, and camping. Over the last three years since the injury I have missed the sense of competition, and the camaraderie of teammates, but I have learned acceptance and learned that there are things in life that we cannot control.

Cancun, Mexico

It was now our senior year, we had waited four years for this spring vacation that we would be spending in Cancun, Mexico. Ever since we had heard the stories from the seniors that had gone on the same voyage the three years prior. It was now our turn to surrender all inhibitions in the perfect tropical climate, and rich festive atmosphere of Gulf of Mexico.

It wasn't until three o'clock in the morning that we arrived at our hotel, The Cancun Beach Hotel and Resort, after a long anxious flight that had been delayed from Logan International Airport in Boston, Massachusetts due to the unexpectedly bad weather in April had knocked down a satellite. We had all worked many hours serving tables, landscaping, telemarketing, or doing whatever other odd job to earn money for the trip, so we immediately went downtown to the clubs. Amidst a seventy degree night surrounded by palm trees, a far contrast from the slushy roads and bitter cold of New Hampshire, we immediately went to the clubs where we were overwhelmed by the chaos and excitement of this place. Like every other night we stayed out all night dancing and drinking, a privilege of being eighteen in Mexico.

The days, that started no earlier than noon unless you decided to stay up the entire night, were filled with lounging at the pool-bar or on the beach. It felt almost surreal, as if we were in paradise. It was an eighteen year-old American's dream to have so much freedom and recreation surrounding them. We filled the days with swimming amidst the warm Gulf of Mexico, and the nights with partying at some of the world's most famous nightclubs. Events were constantly going around us, we snorkeled, went on a booze cruise, bungee-jumped, and parasailed.

Every second of every day was enjoyable. It was hard to return home from such fun, but we all needed our own beds, our own town, and our family and friends back home. The thirty of us that went down there perhaps had the most fun that we will ever experience again. It is my plan to return there next spring break to attempt to duplicate the incredible time I had there.

Athletic Injury

Draft 2

Ryan Corlis Trombly

For the last two weeks of what had seem to be an endless summer vacation I had strenuously struggled through three-mile runs, being pushed around, and incessant practices to secure a position on the my high school's varsity soccer team. The fact that it all paid off and I now would be playing alongside all the seniors and juniors that I had looked up to the year prior left me with one huge sense of accomplishment. I would now have to deal with the stressful schedule of varsity soccer practices and games nearly everyday for the next two and half months coupled with the schoolwork brought about by my sophomore year in high school; including dreaded Geometry, and even more dreaded Biology. It all didn't matter though I was now part of Manchester-Central High School's varsity soccer team.

My first time playing on the varsity team was a friendly scrimmage against a lower division high school and was supposed to be a helpful warm-up before the real season begun. The scrimmage was on a cool overcast day on the first day of September (the last day of that endless summer vacation), before the brisk winds of autumn had rolled in. It was early in the morning, and the grass was still damp from the dew that had been left behind by the night before. As I walked out on the field to prepare for the game my stomach turned with anxiety, not the anxiety caused by nervousness but rather anticipation. This was my favorite time of the year, when the leaves begin to foliate in southern New Hampshire and the foreboding winter that lay ahead started to make its presence known. I glanced around trying to take my mind off the approaching challenge savoring my surroundings; the grass cushioning my hurried steps, the new smell of smoke flowing from nearby chimneys, and the cool breeze that chilled my temperate body.

"Bring it in!" my coach vehemently yelled from the sideline as we all quickly ran to huddle around him. While he ran threw the names of my teammates and the positions they would be playing I thought to myself where is the best place on the bench to sit. "Ryan, you go in at striker," I couldn't believe I would be starting, but I just figured he wanted me to gain some more experience, and to be honest this would probably be a majority of the playing time I would see during the upcoming season.

The bell whistled and the game began, after running around the field at a hectic pace my throat stung as I gasped for the cold air that filled my overheated body as it often did in this weather. Wanting to immediately impress my coach and fellow teammates I put forth my fullest effort as I concentrated on not screwing up and hustling constantly, but not even ten minutes into the game my prior efforts and future goals were abruptly ended by the goalie of the opposing team.

The ball had traveled over several defenders heads and right to my feet as I streamed towards the oppositions goal, quickly running I flew by the final defender and towards the goalie as my mind went blank and gut instinct took over. The goalie sprinted forth from his position to make one last attempt at protecting his net. Directly at one another we ran with utterly different ideas of what was to now occur. Simultaneously as I stiffly planted my left leg and forcefully swung my right to send the ball far into the back of the net the goalie lunged out at me throwing his shoulder into my extended knee snapping it backwards against momentum and hyper extending it. I lied face down in the grass as intense pain surged threw my leg as teammates, opponents, and coaches ran out to assist me aware of the severity due to just witnessing the incident.

I was urgently rushed to the Lahey-Hitcock Clinic, but not after a few excruciating mishaps when I forced to put weight on my knee only to see it completely give out on me. In the pristine waiting room I literally sat in the wheelchair they had given me at the door and sobbed, reflecting on the many days as a kid growing up running about everywhere and the satisfaction that sports had brought to my life that would now not be there. After examining x-rays and evaluating the condition of my knee Dr. Vailas, a talented orthopedic surgeon, scheduled my surgery for the following morning that was supposed to be my first day of my sophomore year. Rather than fraternizing with friends in the hallways and sitting threw classes that now seemed not so bad, I would be on an operating table for six hours, unconscious.

My knee had been hyper extended so badly that I tore two ligaments, snapped two tendons, tore cartilage, and fractured my fibula. Later the doctor and physical therapists would tell me that the only time they saw knee injuries like my case was in car accidents over thirty-miles per hour, which wasn't a great fact to know. Needless to say my competitive athletic career was now over, something that was quite a hard adjustment due to the large role athletics had played in my life.

The next four months were filled with attempting to catch up with my schoolwork as I crutched around a rather large school with a lot of stairs, and with daily rehabilitation sessions with a personal physical therapist for one and half hours a day following school. The sessions were filled with excruciating exercises that were meant to strengthen my knee that had diminished to literally skin and bones. I absolutely dreaded the short drive down to the clinic, and the moments in the shower when my leg would be unwrapped and the horrors of my injury were revealed. After months of this disheartening routine I was left with a little more than eighty percent of the strength that me knee had before this unfortunate incident, and that was the best it would ever be.

Although the reality of my situation was difficult to deal with at the time and for a time after it was an adjustment that I forced to make. Sports were my release, my chance to escape from the hassles of everyday life and now that aspect of my life was just gone. Rather than playing competitive sports my energy was focused to recreational activities, such as playing on my church's CYO team and winning a state championship, going snowboarding all over New Hampshire, Vermont, and Maine, along with backpacking, camping, and flyfishing in the White Mountains whenever the chance arose. Over the last three years since the injury I have missed the sense of competition, the release sports provided me, and the camaraderie of a team, but I have learned that there are things in life that we cannot control.

Good Times Bad Times

Draft 3

Ryan Corlis Trombly

Friday August 31, 1997

Two weeks of hell have finally paid off. Double sessions really wiped me out, one practice a day is hard enough. Three-mile runs under twenty minutes, never ending drills of sprinting and dribbling, my legs felt as if they'd fall off, my lungs felt like they'd burst, and my back was so damn soar that on several mornings I felt as if it might snap under the weight of my body when I first stood up from bed. Well that's a little much, but I couldn't believe how much this has taken out of me. It All Doesn't Matter Though . . . I made the varsity team for Manchester High School—Central's varsity soccer team, as a sophomore, and that's all that matters right now, it all paid off! My parents and I celebrated by going to Shorty's, as we know my favorite restaurant, where I was treated to barbecue quesadillas, and I even got fried ice cream, what an added bonus! I can say they'd probably brought me out and spoiled me more if I hadn't made the team. My sophomore year starts Tuesday and our first scrimmage is against Bow on Monday. They should be awful. Sophomore year should be some good times.

Tuesday September 4, 1997

Life has never been worse. The scrimmage against Bow was yesterday, and I was absolutely correct, they sucked, we beat them 6 to 1. Unfortunately, I missed almost the entire game. Never have I ever been more excited for a game before as the Calen, Noce, and the rest of the upperclassmen ranked on me for having such skinny legs, and for being one of the only two sophomores on the team, and also for the familiarity I would have with the splinters from the worn wooden benches I would be riding. But guess what I started, something that was probably an even bigger indication that I'd see no playing time because the game didn't matter. Well I started and not even three minutes into the game I was taken out. By the goalie. I rushed to the net as he rushed at me, I could of swore that I'd score a goal as I lined up to kick the ball into the back of the net, something I was infamous for doing last year on junior varsity. It didn't work out that way though at all, rather than cheering and excitement I was left with pain, excruciating pain. The goalie took me out. I laid on the ground as the pain, more pain than I ever care to feel again ran through my body, rushed through my body not just my knee that had just been snapped completely the other way: I couldn't catch my breath, the goalie's horror on his face, the noise it made, the scared faces of the people in the crowd (no one clapped), my mother cried, my father lost his stoicism . . . I knew how serious it was. I actually sobbed in the waiting room, I tried not to, but I knew. It took the doctor only ten minutes to describe everything that I would need to know: torn ACL, LCL, PCL; snapped tendons, fractured fibula, torn cartilage, and perhaps nerve damage, "This is a bad one," as he said. GREAT! Rather than seeing my friends at school and sitting through classes waiting for soccer practice I was laid out unconscious on an operating table. Good news no nerve damage, bad news I'll never be able to play competitive sports again and I'll need about three more months of rehab. These are now some pretty damn bad times.

Wednesday, October 23, 1998

Life just isn't good right now. The only thing I have to look forward to are the percocets that get me through the day and the cigarettes that I swore I'd never smoke. Its hard to take showers, not because of the obvious reasons, but because the scars, and the fact that all the muscle in my leg has deteriorated. I've lost like fifteen pounds, the pain killers ruin my appetite. School has been a little harder that I thought, Biology and Geometry are impossible and I just don't have the enthusiasm for school. I need to catch up. My armpits hurt more than my knee for Christ sakes, these crutches are torture. The only time I go out is to the Football games every Friday, where some drunk kid usually falls into me causing me to put weight on my knee, causing intense unneeded pain. Besides that I relax in my house playing videogames, watching movies, and making up excuses for why I need more percocet to mom so she'd get more from the pharmacist. Tomorrow in physical therapy is the first day they're really going to work my knee, GREAT, as if they don't hurt me enough. I have to say its not so bad when Linda, the cute one, is the one inflicting the pain. All the same I'm sick and tired of going to rehab for two hours of the day as the nice days slip away into the wintery kind that will brighten me up even more.

Thursday January 11, 1998

Today my knee was tested in some scary looking machine for strength; compared to my right knee my injured left knee was at sixty-seven percent strength. It will get a little stronger but not much. I've lost a total of twenty pounds, and I'm now limited to vicadin, a lesser strength pain killer, that they only gave me because I still complained of intense pain that isn't so intense. School's going alright, could be certainly better, my parent are a little disappointed. One thing that I think is funny though is the fact that not too many of my teammates have the same camaraderie that they used to show me. OH Well, I've met quite a lot of people since I lost my jock status. Now that I'll no longer need crutches it's nice even to walk, at least I can walk. I'm just ecstatic that two hours a day, five days a week, won't be spent in a clinic where I'd be subjected to having my scars rubbed so they wouldn't anchor the skin, drills of endless balancing, having my knee bended past the point it had grown to allow, and strenuous sessions of exerting all my might on weight machines. Things in my life have really changed, it's hard to watch the younger kids running around without a care in the world, I was once the same as them.

Sunday March 26, 2000

I know it's been a long-ass time since I've written about my knee injury, but I don't think its been until now that I could really truly deal with the after affects of my knee injury. I know a lot of people have knee injuries, and it seems like once a week I'm hearing someone else's story about how they hurt their knee, usually concluding in a torn ACL or torn cartilage. These people are always going on and on until I simply tell them the severity of my injury and show them some battle scars, at which time they say ohhhh, that's really bad. It's not that I don't feel for these people, don't get me wrong it's just that my injury was damn awful. Today after watching my old friends from Central's varsity basketball team, that I also had played for my freshman year and would have started on this year, win the class L State Championship, it was hard to deal with. I forgot how much sports meant to me until today and it was hard, even though I starred on this year's St. Catherine CYO league team and had too won a state championship it wasn't the same. These were the same kids I had played with only a few years ago, sharing laughs, suicides, and victories that now acted like I didn't exist because I was no longer a "jock." The school and town congratulated and honored these kids, these kids I could have been a part of. We all shared the same goal to win the class L New Hampshire State championship, and they did it without me, without even the thought of me. Unfortunate occurrences happen in life that we can not control. The way in which we deal with these occurrences are what determine our character.

I am what I am

Freewrite

Ryan Corlis Trombly

Have you ever seen the movie, *My Blue Heaven,* well that's my neighborhood See spot run down the street as fathers mow their impeccable green lawns and mothers intently watch their young gregarious children run about and scream with joy The Tremblays, the Creamers, the Guitobonis, the Stems all waving to one another with more excitement than a child's first trip to Disney World Growing up I never knew any different lifestyle than that of my own, Caucasian spoiled kids; with fresh smelling homes, clean clothes, gigantic baseball card collections, whatever new computer game system that was out that year, privileged is what they call it As the years gain on me though and the children aged and the parents aged, and the sweet innocence of children gained tarnish from evil encounters my family, my friends families, all families changed I wasn't familiar with the word dysfunction until I was about twelve and I heard It on a comedic television show I didn't truly know the word's full meaning until I was old enough to recognize dysfunction itself When your young you think that everything is wonderful and it will never change, and as the years gain and things do tragically change and the world that you thought was is revealed to be something utterly different, life sucks—Husbands can only stay at work for so long avoiding their wives that they can no longer identify with, wives can no longer find satisfaction in their lives as secondary money earners or housewives, children acquire a hatred for time spent with their dad whose grumpy due to being "overworked" and mom whose aloof because she took too many milligrams of prozac and drank too many mudslides As the paint on the houses fades, and the grass turns from fresh, vibrant green to dry, dull yellows and browns, and the Youngs, the McGoverns, and the Browns no longer wave as you pace by their homes The facade is torn away by the hands of time and the lives of "Suburbia" fade.

Sketches of Evaluation

Draft 4

Ryan Corlis Trombly

Who am I? To answer this question I came to the conclusion that it would be best to examine my life at glance, and then to take a closer look at the events of my life that determined who I am, and finally I examined who I have become. With each one I feel you can get a better sense of who exactly it is that I am. My story is not extraordinary, but it is my own. Here is the life I lead, here is how I got to where I am, here is my upbringing, here are my feelings, here are my thoughts, here this is who I am.

I. At a Glance

Have you ever seen the movie *My Blue Heaven,* well my neighborhood looks identical. The constant hum of lawnmowers as fathers tend to their impeccable lawns and the constant rumble of laughter as the mothers attentively watched over their young gregarious children as they scurry about aimlessly. Growing up I never knew any other lifestyle but my own: spoiled children with fresh smelling homes, enormous lawns, clean matching clothes, gigantic boxes full of baseball cards, the latest video game system. Privileged is what they call it.

As the years gained, and the children aged and the parents aged, and the shimmering innocence grew tarnished, my family, my friends families, all families changed. I wasn't familiar with the word dysfunction until I was about twelve and I heard it on a sketch comedy television show. I didn't truly understand the word dysfunction until I began to experience It first-hand. When your young you think everything is wonderful and it will never change, but as the height measurements on the basement door rose, and the greatness of puberty set in my world came crashing down as I became aware of my surroundings for the first time. Communication is lost, and understanding is brushed aside.

Husbands can only stay at work for so long avoiding their wives that they can no longer identify with, wives can no longer deal with their lives as secondary money-earners or housewives. Children acquire a hatred for time spent with their dad who's always grumpy from being "overworked" and mom who's aloof because she took too many milligrams of prozac and had one too many mudslides. Left to rely on one's self for motivation and moral support. The paint on the house fades, the grass turns from vibrant, fresh green to dull, dry yellows and browns. The facade is torn away by the hands of time, the robust laughter and beautiful innocence is blown away by the wind, and once cordial smiles turn to stern stares.

II. A Closer Look

Born to a hard working farm boy from New Hampshire
and a long dark-haired girl from South Carolina,
I never cried.
They say you'd never seen a fatter baby,
I always laughed

—they didn't let me go to the funeral,
"I like to go swimming with bow-legged women so I can
dive between their knees," he'd say with charm.
Only five years I had with him, but he's the person I most
remember,
I was even blessed with his quirky name, Corlis.
A farmer, a kind neighbor, a loving husband, a hard
worker, a great father, and the best grandfather.
He lived a simple life, but he lived his life.
—he is my character, strength, morals, and pride.

I cried everyday of kindergarten, they sent me to
readiness,
I did the same thing.
I would wake up crying, and scurry to the security of my
parents warm bed through the dark cold of the night.
I was horrified of death,
I sucked my thumb incessantly, the orthodontist bill must
have been high.
—I grew out of this stage

Barefoot and free my youth was filled with slivers.

A rambunctious boy I was, always shy around those not familiar.
Always wore a white tee-shirt to show the efforts of my day.
Woke with the dew, slept with the chirping crickets.
Knew no better, knew no worse, this was my innocence.
—These days are gone

First kiss, cheesy Friday night dances, growing pains, camp in the summer, popularity, confusion, making the team, unpopularity, zits, hormones, hair, a breath of reality, no freedom, bicycles, sweaty palms, bad decisions, boredom.
If I only knew, this was my puberty.
—I am glad these years are gone

High school, perhaps four years of my greatest personal development:
growth and maturity, understanding and acceptance, frustration and strength.
The wrong step, a fall from grace, overcoming.
Nothing like the first time I drove a car alone, the bonfires on Tower Hill Road, SATs, Doc Hussey, Central Pride, "keggers," friends, all the best firsts.
It all went too soon, my childhood, my adolescence, my teenage years: the times, regrets, stories, laughs, hard times.
—New obstacles each day, old memories far away.

And on I go.

III. Examining Now

"It is easy in the world to live after the world's opinion; it is easy in solitude to live after our own; but the great man is he who in the midst of the crowd keeps with perfect sweetness the independence of solitude."

Ralph Waldo Emerson, *Self Reliance*

This was my senior quote, when I first read this essay by Emerson this line stuck out like a soar thumb. Threw my life and after many experiences and interactions I came to really truly understand the meaning of these words. It is important to rely on one's own opinion and thoughts, while others hold their own. Although it may be easier to agree and conform to the ideas of a crowd, to be a true person is to be a non-conformist with the strength and confidence of believing and relying on one's self. Here is who I have become and who I want to become, this is where I have led myself, this is the life I created, this is my own work.

My mood depends on the weather,
I need the sun to shine.
It is probably best to leave me alone on a cloudy day.
I love to be alone.
Don't get me wrong I love the company of friends.

My father is a "workaholic," as my mother describes him.
I call him "Tommy-Boy"
Nearly no married couples I know are happy with each other.
I want to have five children; three boys, two girls.
My parents never let me have a dog, I'll probably raise a kennel of them.

As a child I didn't wear shoes regularly until I was five and went to school.
I never take off my shoes now; sometimes I sleep in them.
Maps were my true love,
I want to see the world, live amongst foreign peoples and feel their culture.
A honeymoon to Bermuda and a retirement vacation to England will probably be the extent of my travels.

The Nobel Peace Prize is my goal in life,
I want to find a cure.
Every profession from lumberjack to politician has at one time appealed to me,
I don't want to spend my life in school.
Poor would be the last thing I'd want to be.

Every morning when I wake up I am oblivious to where I am,

I don't sleep very well.
After a bite of a meal that looks delicious, I feel full,
I don't have the best eating habits.
Weight is just a number, I hate when people tell me I'm skinny, would they tell a person that their fat with such ease.

Some people tell me I'm a great listener, others say I never listen,
I have selective hearing.
Everyone tells me I'm random,
I am constantly thinking.
My mind torments me at times, especially at 4:00 am on a Tuesday night when I can't sleep.

People say I'm stubborn,
I just have my own opinions.
Some say that I'm too intense,
I just have places I want to go in life.
Life is too short to be complacent.

The forest is where I feel most at home,
I love white birch trees, and foliage.
Wool is my favorite fabric, I feel it fits all occasions,
I love when the sunbeams glisten through the leaves.
Nothing is more comfortable then wrapping up in blankets during the winter.

A log cabin in northern Vermont is where I'd love to spend my life,
I'll probably own a colonial in a housing development on Long Island.
When I grow up I'd like to have a career that interests me,
I'll get bored with any profession that I do.
All I want is a life without regrets.

Love and happiness is all I want.
I have a hard time being away from Caitrin.
We've always been friends; we grew up together.
I often wonder if my life will be filled with happiness,
No one loves me more than her.

My grandfather is the biggest influence in my life,
I have no idea what death is like; it frightens me, I'm not religious.
He instilled in me character, strength, morals, and pride.
I live to breath air, to run through grass, to scream at the top of my lungs.
Still to this day I have yet to visit my grandfather's gravesite.

I

Rain

Draft 1

Jessica Burns

She stared out that screen the piece of glass that separated her from the miracle she was young and sad he was young and free the rain slipping like her tears the slamming of the thunder like her fathers slamming of her all those years like her mothers slamming of her like the worlds slamming of her into a cold wall with each pound she remembered with each pound she fell deeper and deeper missing the miracle the miracle the miracle of him and her and her and him the bird the keeper could she could she crack that door could she break that glass could she cut through that screen could she anymore could she just let him in a little more oh god oh god why was she so afraid he was such a miracle that day that day in the rain.

Personal Snapshot

Alexis Krech

The hospital stunk. They had a very recognizable odor. There was this unmistakable smell of disinfectant bleach and sick people.

I laid flat on my back in a hospital bed. The only thing that ran through my mind is how much I wanted to get up and walk out. I felt trapped, in a locked cage. The doctors kept coming in and asking me questions, an endless stream of the same questions. They tried to be nice and gave me medical explanations of what they were going to do, but it was just a blur of words that made no sense to me.

Later, they put a tube in my nose that led down to my stomach. The uncompassionate nurses jammed an IV into my hand, all the while, pretending I wasn't even human. Then they came back, ripping out the first nose tube and replacing it with another. Under normal circumstances it would have been very painful, but I felt no pain and said nothing. I just lay there motionless like a dummy.

I was wheeled from room to room through different corridors that were suspiciously empty of people. I studied the passing lights and ceiling, a faint yellow then cheesy white paneling. The nurses wheeling me around would whisper to each other about me as if I couldn't hear them.

In my semi-conscious state they finally put me in my own room. I didn't care. I just wanted all the doctors and nurses to leave me alone. Every hour they would predictably return to poke and prod me like I was an animal. Shivering and cold, beads of a cold sweat ran down my face. I wanted more blankets, but they won't give me any more, so I just suffered quietly.

Somehow, I finally drifted off to sleep. I learned to ignore everyone that came into my room. As I fell into a deep sleep, I could barely hear my sister and mom in the background, lightly crying. I wanted to reach my hand out to them, to hold them, and say sorry.

Regurgitated, Half Digested Mouse Surprise

Joe Bartlett

Recipe History

Almost everyone who is anyone has heard about the day when Earl met Joe and the fourth worst smell known to man came into existence. Months of research and experimentation have led to the discovery of this recipe, which allows anyone to recreate this momentous occasion in a special young man's life. It all happened one beautiful October day in a fall color filled valley in southern Ohio. A young man named Joe was volunteering for the first time at the Raptor (bird of prey) Rehabilitation Center. A day of fun filled excitement was nearing its end when Joe was presented with the opportunity to hold a turkey vulture name Earl, the rest of the story soon went down in the annals of history. In fact four definitive writings were composed on the subject in a college English class documenting the tale. The film rights to the story were purchased by the same people who brought you **When Animals Decide not to Attack but do Really Incredibly Nasty Things to Unsuspecting Humans Who Then Look Quite Surprised and Often Vomit Parts I, II, and VII.** Due to the immense number of letters received after our first publication of this recipe, we at *Weird Recipes for Weird People* had an interview with the one they call Joe and his comments are found after the recipe.

Prep time: 30 seconds

Ingredients:

1 14-year-old Turkey Vulture named Earl

1 17-year-old male volunteer named Joe

1 leather insulated right-handed glove, which promptly ends at the wrist

1 bare particularly un-acid proof forearm

4 oz. can incredibly, disgustingly, horribly, vomit inducing, retina burning, special chunky mouse sauce

1 half-digested mouse, preferably white with at least two legs missing

2 oz. the fourth worst smell known to man (see page 9)

1 cup pain comparable to childbirth (see page 10)

Place the heavy insulated glove onto the 17 year old male volunteer named Joe's right hand and make sure that the glove promptly ends at his wrists exposing several inches of the particularly un-acid proof forearm. Now perch the 14-year-old Turkey Vulture named Earl onto the glove. Make a guttural, gurgling, choking noise and combine the special chunky mouse sauce, the half-digested mouse, the cup of pain and spread over the bare un-acid proof forearm to form a thick coating. Finally take the 4th worst smell known to man and spread over the upper lip of the 17-year-old male and cause him to deeply inhale.

Makes 1 serving

Hello readers, my name is Joe Bartlett and by now most of you probably already know my story but I would like to share some of the things I learned from this experience. Aside from discovering the fourth worst smell known to man and the pain comparable to childbirth, I now know that the events of that day have had a profound affect on my life. First of all, it was an incredibly beautiful day, one of those that forever sticks in your mind because everything seemed so perfect. I was standing with my back to a national scenic river with a covered bridge over it, surrounded by the oranges and reds of fall, a beautiful and majestic bird on my arm, and I knew this was a special moment. Then the bird vomited on my arm and it made me famous, but that really isn't the most important part of the day. As much as I like my new house and my two BMW's, I owe much more than that to Earl. I learned to respect nature that day. I had always wanted to study the environment but my experience with Earl taught me something more. The voluateers at Raptor always called it an education moment whenever a bird poops on the floor during a demonstration, but I think that the vomit on my arm was the biggest educational moment of all. I experienced nature and I wished that others could have that same experience. With this new recipe, anyone can have the raw unbridled fury of nature, so I recommend that everyone make the Regurgitated, Half Dead Mouse Surprise and make it as often as possible. Also, don't forget to see my movie and read my book, both should be out by Christmas, and if you have a little one who is too young to read, a line of clothes and action figures will be on the shelves soon. I would like to take this opportunity to thank Earl for making all of this possible, but mostly I would like to thank you, yes you, the sick disgusting people who actually make this recipe and buy my shameless products.

Sincerely,

Joe Bartlett

Rice Girl

Jennifer

I am what I am. I'm an American citizen born in California. Two days after New Years' eve in 1982, a set of twins is born to a mother who came to United States 2 years ago. Her fifteen months son is at home with his babysitter safe sleeping in his bed. Her husband is right next to her while she gives birth. One came out the way babies usually did, and the other one she had to get C-section on. She names her new set of babies Tiffany and Jennifer.

I can't go back to my country because America is my country. I'm Asian. I'm Vietnamese. My mom is quarter Chinese. So, technically, I have a little Chinese in me, too.

White rice is what I eat everyday, but who says eating healthy is bad for you. I don't have to eat rice everyday. The short, brown hair girl approached my group of friends and I as we were eating our lunch. She saw me eating crispy, golden fries. She suddenly asked if I had to eat rice with everything since my other friend, Joyce, who happened to be Chinese, did.

No, I don't have small eyes. And they're not slanted as you think all Asians have. No, even if I do have small eyes, I see everything fully, not in halves. The boy looks at me. He starts to squint one way and another. His small, pale hands quickly move to his huge, round, blue eyes. Then with a quick hand movement pulled the skin around his eyes up and asks how come my eyes aren't like that.

I like listening to Vietnamese music. So peaceful and quiet like being out on the countryside. It helps keep the heritage I never knew in me. It teaches me more Vietnamese words and phrases. My friend got a ride home with my dad and I in our Honda Passport. My dad was listening to his Vietnamese music. All of a sudden I hear a laugh. What's so funny? Oh, the music you're listening to. I can't understand a thing and it sounds funny. Nothing's funny about it. You just don't understand the meaning to it.

I like speaking Vietnamese. No, when I'm speaking Vietnamese with my friends, I'm not talking about you. Can you guys stop talking like that? I can't understand a thing that is being said. Don't worry; it's not about you. She was asking me something she couldn't explain in English.

I have a lot of friends that are different races. My best friends include: Laos, Black, Chinese, and Caucasian. I grew up all over east coast. I moved around the country, never satisfied with one place. No, I'm not an army kid. From sunny California to cold Utah. From Utah to dirty Philadelphia. Proceed to Detroit. Then to quiet Vermont. I'm not a Vermont native. Four years has passed since I've laid claims to stay here.

I like reading thick, intriguing books. I also like reading the newspaper, too. Sunday mornings I always looked forward to. I run and grab the comic section first. Oh, how I love reading the comics and laughing out loud. The colorful pictures were a sight. I need more money. For what? To get myself a new set of books to read. There's nothing wrong with that. It helps enhance my knowledge, let alone helps me become well educated. Middle school I read a lot. I ended up with straight A's, and a 4.0 GPA.

I love to draw. My room is wearing my drawings. Art exam, draw a scene from a mountain. Wow that is really good. I love the shading to it. May I keep it to show to my next class? Okay. Make your own comics. My friend runs up to me. She tells me she just saw one of my drawings. Really good work. She told me I could make a career out of it.

Fashion is my scene. I don't care what you have to say about the way I dress. What is that? An apron? Are you cooking? Yeah I am. And you're my first course. Stares. Glances. How odd. Yeah, I'm wearing a skirt with a pair of black pants underneath. Statement, yes. Looks good, indeed.

Why dress the same as everybody else?

I have to stick out from everybody else. I like wearing color contacts. Okay take this pair of contacts and place it between your forefinger. Now take your thumb and your middle finger and spread apart your eyelids. Now place your contact in. Tears streamed down my face like water running from the faucet. It stung. Blink. Blink.

Freak! You look like one with those green contacts you're wearing. And it doesn't go with your hair color. Either those contacts go or your hair color goes. Pick. It doesn't mean that I want to be somebody else or that I'm afraid of what I am. It shows I like to experiment with things that make me different or look different. I like dyeing my hair different colors, too.

Wow. That's a really nice color. Red highlights. Stands out. Hmm, I see blonde too. It looks like fall. Very berry! Oh and look, your natural color is there too. Makes you look healthy with that glow on your skin.

I am a twin. Do we look alike? No. Tiffany. No, I'm Jennifer. Tiffany is my sister. Oh right. You two look alike I get mixed up. You two don't look anything alike. Than how do people get us mixed up?

I'm an individual. I'm dependent. I don't like people spending too much money on me. I don't want to seem like I'm using them. Here let me pay for that. No, no, it's okay. I have money. Yeah and so do I. Save your money for something really useful. Something you will need.

I like learning things on my own. I looked through the book. Oh, okay. I get it now. It makes more sense. I wish I knew this before.

I do things on my own, too. Here, have your brother put this desk up for you. Ha. Ha. Funny. It will take him hours or days before he gets it up. Here I can do it myself.

The brown, three shelves bookshelf. It's still standing after four years of putting it up. What a good job I did. I'm proud of it. It's also still in good condition.

I like to travel. It's fun to see new places. Experience the feel to the city or country. I stepped off the plane into the hot humid surroundings. I looked around. Wow. I made the 36 hours plane ride. I am now on the other side of the world.

I get into a lot of trouble. In the end, it's all worth it. My good grades erases and replaces the troubles I get myself into. The pager went off and still no phone calls. It's midnight. Around four in the morning I get into the house. I get a lecture, but the next day it's okay. It's been forgotten.

I am me. I am a person. I am a person with feelings. I am a human being with mistakes. I am here to accomplish my goals with my life and fulfill my dreams. I am here.

Unfinished Nails

Adam Effler

In elementary school, it was a common occurrence for students to be called out of class to serve a funeral at the nearby church. I attended a private, catholic school where serving wasn't just requested of you. It was "expected of you as your duty to God." If I don't feel comfortable serving, will I go to hell? Many kids became anxious upon request.

I had always enjoyed serving funerals. They were always the same. No surprises. I was more enlightened by the feeling of sorrow that filled a church funeral than by the sorrow that filled me while having to sit through another boring religion class. My senses heightened twice over while listening to the eloquence of a family member speak in honor of the deceased. The feeling was really there. Death was a reality, not just a misconstrued thought written in "Jesus, yesterday and today", the fifth grade religion text.

So it happened that three of my classmates and I were asked to serve one day in the fall of 1992. I left with a smile on my face, undoubtedly pissing off Mrs. Mathis. Mrs. Mathis was one of those teachers who enjoy their job partly because they get to order little kids around. She never truly liked how mobile I was. My three friends begged not to have to go. Their antagonism had zero affect, and so we left, crossing the parking lot towards the church. After Eric, Julie, Sarah, and I put on our robes and cross necklaces, we continued to set up for mass. I was instructed to get the incense pan ready. I remember how excited I was for this job because there was no smell that I liked more than that of incense.

The incense pan dangled from a decorative copper chain and hung from a stand located at the rear entrance of the church. From this entrance I was able to gaze out into the church. I was astonished to see that there were eight priests helping with the service. This was exceptionally strange because attendance was minimal. The lady who had died seemed to have a decent sized family but few friends. I figured that the priests came upon special request. Regardless, they congregated, forming a mass of white cloth at the head of the church. Each priest had his own intricately embroidered shawl with dangling tassels, which was draped perfectly over his shoulders. The family stood clad in black from the neck down. The room consisted entirely of youthful faces, the next generation of the deceased. Many of her friends and family must have died off

The service continued to run as normal. Often, families choose to have a short funeral to lessen the burden that it inflicts on them. This one was short. They're always the same. After a quick processional the eldest son, knowing his role and playing just fine, stood to the podium and gave his speech. The speech was more focused on the memories of the lady with her friends than on the lady as an individual. As I watched tears pour buckets down the face of her family, it quickly became apparent to me that her family mourned for the death of a generation. She was the last.

After the speech, I followed the priest, with the incense burner, to the casket. I watched as he swung it back and forth in front of the big wooden box, never truly knowing what he was doing. I always just figured that it was a blessing. The mass was now over and all of us sewers followed the eight priests back down the isle to the front church entrance. The casket soon followed. And behind the casket followed the family. We stood to the side as the pallbearers carried the casket right by us. Suddenly, a loud crack could be heard echoing throughout the church.

Within seconds, the bottom of the casket gave way in front of the eight priests, four alter sewers, and entire family. I looked down to see the old, dead lady smack to the floor and roll over. It looked painful, even for a dead person. There is always those first few seconds in a disaster where no one reacts because of disbelief. For those first seconds I saw pure beauty. Her body had fallen so that her head was turned our way. Her face was content. Maybe it was the makeup but she seemed to be smiling in my direction. My classmates turned away for those quick seconds while I peered deeply into the face of the dead woman. Her crooked, eerie smile sent chills down my spine but it didn't matter because I felt something real. Death was beautiful for those seconds. Her hair was dyed brown, but had a blue tint. It reminded me of my own grandma and my cousins from down south. They would say "Gramma. Yall's hair's blue!" I now knew of a characteristic that may or may not have been defining in this woman's personality. I read deeper than usual. Mass wasn't the same that day. Life wasn't the same that day.

I looked up at the family, expecting to hear shrieks of pain and anguish at having to see such a thing happen to their dearest. They never came. People were not at all disheartened. In fact, the cries ceased. Eyes widened. It felt like time had stopped, bringing everything and everyone in the room to a halt. I saw a few family members fill in the gaps of the people standing around the scene just so they could get a glimpse, a last glimpse. Did they see what I had seen? To this day, I believe that the family gained closure from seeing her face one last time. I know that I did.

The palm bearers, in an attempt to make things all right, lowered the casket top back over the body. "What is the rush?" I thought. I remember how very bothered I was to see them decide to act so rashly. Sure it was a disaster, but this was the very same lady that everyone had been honoring for the last hour. Her arm hung out from the bottom of the box on the left, with hands half clenched. The weight of the box was resting just below her wrist and seemed to be crushing her arm. It looked painful, even for a dead person. The pallbearers tried pushing her arm under the box like someone stuffs their last shirt into a suitcase just before zipping it closed. I was sickened. I was compelled to stop them but already knew that it wasn't my place to step in. I looked up at the pallbearers as they glared down at the lady. Their faces displayed a feeling of compassion and they did not know that they were doing wrong. The priests stood still, shocked by something they had probably never seen happen. I was left breathless, questioning my own feelings, and trapped in a scene which provided few answers.

The Colors That Changed My Perspective

Lindsay Geoghegan

A foreign but pleasing smell surrounded me the first time I jumped off the bus and flew through the large red doors. I learned later that the aroma was that of rich Chinese cooking that seeped through the walls from the restaurant next door. This smell eventually became familiar and even comforting, but not before a lot of adjusting. The halls were long, concrete, and intimidating. Bright orange and yellow pictures of children playing were painted along the sides of the hallway, and glossy tiles covered the floors. The outside of the building was similarly decorated with what appeared to be children's drawings painted on top of a shockingly yellow border. As a child, I can remember passing by this flamboyant asymmetrical building as we drove down the highway; my curiosity ran wild as to what went on inside. So there I was, years later, actually enrolled in this bilingual elementary school in the heart of Boston's China Town.

Monday September 9, 1992
Wyeduc:

We were sitting at our assigned lunch table, a long portable picnic table on wheels. There were fifty of us, sitting rigidly, staring one another face to face. No one said a word, because you were not allowed to. This silence may have seemed awkward to a newcomer, but I was accustomed to it, having been at the Quincy School for five years. Just as I was biting into my chicken patty, I hear a voice from the end of the table attempt to make small talk with the girl sitting next to her. It was the new girl, Lindsay, whose voice that I heard. Instead of responding, in fear of getting reprimanded, the girl sitting next to her smiles politely, then continues to concentrate on her meal. But it was too late. The lunch lady, who everyone referred to as the wicked witch, starts hollering at the top of her lungs, "No talking during lunch!" Before Lindsay knew it, her lunch was swept up in front of her, and she was moved to sit in a private lunchroom all alone. We only had a certain amount of time to scarf down our lunches before we were ordered to whip out our books, and begin reading. Of course, Lindsay had forgotten her book, so she sat in solitaire as everyone else pretended to read.

A new pink cotton dress was the perfect attire for my first day of fourth grade. My hair was freshly cut, and I had ambitious goals set in my mind. I felt as though I was ready to make a change, I was ready to be independent. I had outgrown my previous school, and conveniently told my parents this the same time that the tuition was being raised. The school had a good reputation; its claim to fame was "the best grade school in Boston", but other than that I knew very little about what I would encounter.

I had previously attended a small liberal private school tucked in the rural suburbs of Chestnut Hill. The teachers were supportive and nurturing. The school was predominantly white, so I was one of the crowd. At my new school, I was a distinct minority. In the beginning this was very overwhelming; I felt out of place and all alone. No one was going to comfort me. Students who had it much worse surrounded me. Is there really a need to console a privileged white girl? A mold was formed for me before I had time to form one for myself. I was automatically assumed to be smart, wealthy, and snobby, which I was not. It took time and effort to overcome these stereotypes.

Wednesday October 10, 1992
Wyeduc:

Trying to get my usual seat in the back of the bus, I do a little pushing and shoving of the people in front of me. As I was on my mission, I accidentally knocked Lindsay, book bag and all into one of the front seats. I felt bad, but decided not to apologize because a seat in the front of the bus was her permanent position anyhow. She sat stiffly with her bag tightly fastened to her back; she barely moves an inch during the entire ride. She would stare in awe as we passed the Howard Johnson's, and saw several prostitutes lurking outside of the building. This probably being a sight she had never before witnessed. My friends and I were interested in getting an expression out of her. So one day, my friend, Ambuli, jumped in her face and started singing, "Chris Cross will make ya jump,jump, daddy mac will make ya." She was startled, and let out a small smile, but didn't appear overly amused.

After making several close friends, I decided to do something more to integrate myself into The Josiah Quincy School. I had heard of the dance auditions by word of mouth. The core dance troupe had already been formed; the instructors were only looking for a few additional dancers. A whole row of girls and boys filed down to the cool, damp gym in the basement of the building. Mr. Chan and his daughter lined us up horizontally along the gym floor. We were asked to do a few simple combinations, but nothing too complicated, I think that they were looking for grace and spirit instead of technique. After the auditions, they read aloud a list of those who made the troupe. My heart was beating so forcefully that I felt as though I were going to burst. I was more relieved than excited when I heard that I had been selected to perform as part of the Chinese Fan Dance along with five other girls.

Tuesday, November 1, 1992
Wyeduc:

As we stood quietly on the gym floor, I take a moment to glance down the long row of those who were auditioning. My eyes stop at Lindsay, only because she was standing differently from the others. She was overly poised, looking as though she was at complete attention. Her feet were turned out in what looked like a prima ballerina pose. What was she thinking? I was hoping to get the part of the dragon, so I wasn't concerned with dancing, just simply running around under a giant costume. Lindsay seemed to take everything too seriously; I couldn't refrain from laughing.

These routines have been a part of the school's tradition as long as it has existed. An indescribable sense of pride engulfed me as I danced. When we performed, our vibrant movements highlighted the stage. Whether we were performing for our fellow students or a hospital full of sick elderly, the response from the audience was the same, enthusiastic and supportive. At my final pose in the dance, I would take a momentary view of the crowd, and see large, approving smiles, vigorous applauding, and standing ovations. The Chinese culture is one for which I have always had a tremendous amount of respect and admiration. Being appreciated, and recognized as a member of my new culture was more than rewarding.

The practices were very time consuming. I can remember sitting in the middle of math class at ten in the morning, and our choreographers, the Chan's, would pull us out of class to practice for upcoming performances. I would receive some animosity from other students during moments like these. I can remember boys yelling out, "Oh Lindsay, you're skipping class again to go dance, Huh?" I never took these comments to heart, believing that my experience dancing was more important than multiplication.

Monday, November 7, 1992
Wyeduc:

Maybe it was because I ended up not being chosen as the part of the dragon, but I was in a bad mood that day. So, when the Chan's came to pull Lindsay out of class to practice for the Chinese New Year Festival, I took the opportunity to free my mind of frustration. She was perceived as an angel to others, but personally did not impress me. I called out something about her always missing class. I remember our teacher, Mr. Lopes, giving me a disapproving look, but didn't mention anything, because he didn't care enough.

Mr. Chan, the head instructor, had been teaching dance at the Quincy School for fourteen years. He was a calm and gentle teacher, who I never recall becoming frustrated. He would teach us the moves with ease, using his simple English vocabulary. Then, he left it up to his daughter to perfect us as a team. His daughter, a beautiful and intelligent lady, did not have such an even temper. When we were under her instruction, practices had no time limit; they consisted of repetition until the moves were precise. At times this would be draining but I enjoyed every minute of it.

Our costumes must have been passed down for years but still exemplified their beauty. Getting dressed in the tiny costume room in the back of an old classroom was a thrill in itself. There would be a cluster of girls scurrying to change into brightly colored garments, each portraying a symbol of the specific dance. My costume consisted of a red flowy skirt and of a red and yellow flowered wrap-around shirt. Under the skirt we wore pink bloomers. In our hair, we wore two braided buns with tiny red roses arranged in a circle around each. In our hands, we carried two elaborate fans with pink fringe, which was a necessity to the smoothness of our dance.

We danced to entertain and educate the city of Boston. Although our dances only lasted a matter of four minutes, I saw the impact of our performance in the eyes of our audience, and this gratified me. Although I may have played an insignificant role, I was finally a part of the culture. As I walked out of those red doors for the final time, I could no longer smell the rich Chinese cooking. I had grown accustomed to it, just as I had grown accustomed to a new me.

A Portrait of an Individual

Cover Letter

Jaime Robertson

I have thoroughly enjoyed the process of writing this paper. The idea of a self-study caught my attention from the very start. At first, I felt like there was too much I needed to say in order to portray myself accurately. I started with three snapshots of events that I felt changed my life. Then, I tried a poem format, and felt it needed more explanation. When I integrated the two I was sad to loose the effect of the poem. So, I decided to remove the parts of the poem that I had integrated into the essay and use them both separately. Lastly, I got this feeling that part of this "portrait" was missing and came up with the poem you will find at the end of my paper. The idea for the last piece came from the comments I received from my best friend when I asked her for a description of myself. The three quotes are from my two favorite books. I read them both recently, during a difficult time in my life and found them to be influential. I am pleased with the way this paper turned out, and am confident that it is a true picture of myself.

A Portrait of an Individual

Jaime Roberston

(Three responses to the question "Who am I?")

"There are few things as seemingly untouched by the real world as a child asleep."

— John Irving, *A Widow For One Year*

I am Corporate America
I have a closet full of
black suits
black shoes
and drawers full of hose
I want to be a housewife
with a husband who humors Corporate America
with a closet full of
black suits
black shoes
and fancy ties on a spinning rack
Instead, I go to med school
so I can deliver babies in my spare time
as I shuttle our 2.4 children to and from
dance class
softball practice
soccer
catholic church and private school
I try, but I am imperialistic
materialistic
and I drink low-fat lattes from the Barnes and Noble Star-
bucks down the street
I am Corporate America
but I am waiting to become something else.
I live in a ticky-tacky house
drive an SUV
and wash my hair with Herbal Essence.
I'd use suave if I had to.
I want to be a pregnant waitress
live in a mobile home
drive cross country

and spend my summers in the Rockies
I am corporate America and I am used for my youth
I walk down the street with a boy who wants me to;
tie blue bandanas around our black lab's neck
bake chewy brownies
lie around the house till noon with our beautiful babies
and go to the country club
no worries
But I'm still here because these wants aren't carved in stone
nothing is.
He could go to Harvard
but he's going to Kansas
because he is not Corporate America
And I love him for no reason at all
or because the sky is blue
and the grass green
There is a waterfall at home that I call my place
his arms are my place
I still rub my eyes when I wake up to find him there
I'm only beginning to find places like that here
people and places that can appreciate my many attributes;
I have little ears
I eat pineapples on my pizza
I am blessed with magical friendships
I laugh a lot
I love to roll down the car window and sing at the top of my lungs
I'll never have ulcers
But still, I am Corporate America:
I drive around all day
waiting
at traffic lights that are
red
red
red
Here, they are green.

II.

"Brave means that you accept what happens to you—you just try to make the best of it."

— John Irving, *A Widow For One Year*

I am a product of my own decisions and experience. I have made so many decisions and had so much experience in this short life that I could probably write a book. Yet, just like everyone else out there, there is a picture that I'd like to paint of myself if I had the chance. There are those few choice memories that I believe have made me the individual that I am today: the day my mother died, the day I chose to go to a different high school, the day my friend died, the day I decided to move 1,920 miles away from home, the day I decided who I wanted everyone to see when they looked in my direction.

Three days into my Sophomore year of high school I transferred from Pulaski Academy to Little Rock Central High. My Grandmother still insists that the decision was too large for a 16 year old to make, but it was one of the best decisions I have ever made. I left a predominately white school to enter "the birthplace of desegregation in the south," a class of 85 to graduate with a class of 600, and was privileged to participate in the 40th anniversary of "The Crisis at Central High." I joined the debate team and now know more about Global Warming and Russian Foreign policy than most could even imagine. I met my two greatest companions, experienced more things, and had more opportunity than had ever been presented to me before. Going to Central sent me down one of those "whole new paths" that has helped to shape the person that I am today. Along this path I've run across a few green pastures and a few big boulders have landed in my way. One person that I met at Central High School will always stand out in my mind:

Nilusha Dayananda had HUGE brown eyes, and the greatest laugh I've ever heard. She always painted her toenails red, and wore scarves around her neck. She loved to roll down the windows and sing at the top of her lungs. Her spirit filled the room. It still does. These, along with the horrific picture of the car in the paper, are the first things that come to mind when I think about my friend. I was in Gulf Shores, Alabama when it happened, July 18th, 1998. My dad called that night around 8:30, "there was an accident," he said, "Justin, Robert, and

Nilu were in a car accident . . . Nilu was killed." I didn't go to the funeral. I stayed at the beach. I don't know how I feel about that decision, but I can't change it now. Since the accident, I have spent a lot of time with Nilu's mother. I think watching her deal with the death of her daughter is one of the most terrible things I have ever experienced, but it has helped me in dealing with my mother's death.

To quote Ernest Hemingway, "The world breaks everyone and afterward many are strong at the broken places." I guess you could say I was 'broken' at a very young age. One month alter I was born, my mother was diagnosed with terminal breast cancer. For the next thirteen months my mother struggled to live a full life while battling this terrible disease. She suffered an epileptic seizure on December 25, 1981, my first Christmas. The cancer had spread to her brain. Her health continued to worsen, and my mother died on June 27, 1982. I was fourteen months old. I had no way to express the emptiness that will be with me eternally, and it has shaped the last seventeen years of my life. This is most definitely a tragedy, but it has made me the strong person that I am today.

The loss of my mother at such an early age has impacted every aspect of my life, and Nilu's death simply reminds me how fragile life truly is. I learned early that nothing lasts forever; anything and everything could end in a matter of seconds. I knew this before I knew my ABC's, before I could ride a bike, but I never thought it would happen to a friend, a young friend. These two deaths have helped me to focus on the greater aspects of living. I have the ability to build 'magical' friendships. I live for ice cream in the park, walking barefoot on the beach, building snowmen (and women), and climbing trees. In short, I've learned to stop and smell the tulips (I like them better than roses) and point them out to the ones I love. As a direct result of these tragedies I've conquered, I am a woman with character and more love to give the world than I could ever expect in return. I know how to "plant my own garden, and decorate my own soul." I am determined to live a full life, to extract all I can out of every situation, and to spread the love I have inside around. I suppose this world did manage to 'break' me, but the scars I have developed are worth the price. They have only increased my strength and heightened my sensitivity.

When I am no longer here on this earth, I want a friend of mine to remember me like I remember Nilu. I want someone

I love to remember the girl with freckles in her green eyes, a big smile on her face, and so much love. The girl who made spontaneous decisions to do what seemed to be crazy things. For now, it's all turned out just fine, but I know too well that perhaps it could all end tomorrow.

III.

"If you care about something, you have to protect it- If you're lucky enough to find a way of life you love, you have to find the courage to live it." — John Irving, *A Prayer for Owen Meany*

I am one of Life's beautiful delicates—
pale in the moonlight,
glowing in the sun—
tenderly wrapped in the silk of a spider web,
and fragile to touch.
I am sweet
(like vanilla powder),
clear and pure.
Pale in the moonlight,
glowing in the sun,
I shine—translucent through worries.
I am a guide to light
the footsore and weary,
those battered from life.
I carry on my strong shoulders
soft, satin beauty
waiting to be touched.
I am one of Life's beautiful delicates—
dear and loved,
surrounded by light . . .
Careful, I am delicate.
But I am rough—
always glowing—
sharp and quick.
I am soft but I can cut,
I am power,
I am beauty,
and I am strong.
Pale in the moonlight,
delicate and tender—
I am wonder.

I am an image of everything good,
of everything harsh,
of everything brutal and sharp and cynical—
of all that is pale, is gleaming,
is tender.
I am a delicate beauty.
I am tender,
I am strong.

Interpreting Texts

Topic Proposal

Megan Wells

In our society today, there is a growing amount of teenage children who are being affected by the diseases of Anorexia and Bulimia. Teenage women are especially prone to these diseases because society constantly surrounds them with images of "perfect women" in size zero clothing persuading them that this is how the "ideal woman" should present herself. They see this in a variety of public images, among these is on the covers of major teenage magazines. Teenagers also have access to these magazines wherever they go. They can purchase them through the mail, or at the local convenient store. Even when they are with their parents in the grocery store, these magazines are conveniently placed in the isle of the check out counters, so when waiting in long lines, you can just happen to glance at the covers and instantly be hooked by the beautiful woman on the cover. My argument for this paper is that mainstream society is sexist when it comes to deciding whom they choose to place on the covers of popular teenage magazines.

I am interested in this topic because my family has been personally affected from the images society chooses to show to our young adults. One of my younger sisters has and still is fighting with the disease of Anorexia, and so have some of her fellow classmates. This disease has turned our family upside down. My sister who will be turning 16 in a few months, dropped from a size eight waist to a size zero in a span of just three short months, close to a year ago. Since then she has been fighting the battle to overcome her fears of being "fat." Presently, she has gained a little weight and wears a size one. As bathing suit weather approaches, she fears that she has gained too much weight during this past winter and needs to loose a few pounds before fitting into her tiny bikini. A few months ago she confided in me that pressure from her classmates and today's society has made her go through the torture of starving herself. She also pointed out that some of her friends are in a more drastic state then her. Others have turned bulimic and on top of that take diet pills to loose the little fat they have covering their body. I think this is a complete out rage. This also scares me to death; this is my own sister I am talking about, not just some random person with a problem.

In hopes of writing this paper, I will learn more about this terrible disease and maybe find out ways to help my sister and others to overcome it. When I was in high school, I also remember the pressure to be skinny. During this time, a woman's body is going through so many changes, that one also becomes very emotional. You often take everything that people say to heart. Becoming dangerously skinny at such a young age can really affect a young woman's body in horrible ways. I just pray that my sister never becomes so bad that she has permanent damage to her body. Now that I am in college, I have found that weight is not such a major problem. Yes, one should still be physically active but people frown upon girls that are sticks. I really like this attitude that most college student's posses, they respect you for who you are, and not what you look like.

In the proceeding essays, I will use three different popular teenage magazines to prove my argument. I will first analyze a magazine cover from the popular teenage magazine, "Seventeen". It will most definitely show a beautiful young, skinny woman posing with little clothing covering her tan body. She will probably also be wearing a lot of make up and is in a sexual looking pose.

The second magazine cover I will be defending my argument with is "YM." This stands for Young and Modern. So, are they trying to say that the "new young and modern woman" should be a size zero? This is what I will try to answer when analyzing many of their past and present covers.

The third magazine cover I will analyze will be from, "Us." This magazine talks about all the new hot actors and actresses in the media world. It also features many of the popular supermodels from around the world. You can probably guess what type of people will be on the cover of this magazine, definitely not the plain, normal looking girls of America.

For a secondary source, I think I will interview my younger sister who has the problem with Anorexia. She would be a good resource because she has been personally affected by what society is trying to teach the future generation. She also subscribes to many of the magazines that I have chosen to analyze, so she can tell me her thoughts of the women who are placed on the covers. I also would like to find some sort of text that backs up my argument, perhaps from a magazine article! Not specifically about Magazine covers, but famous and popular women who are way too skinny. I think there is an article in a People's magazine on this subject. It covers popular actresses who have lost obscene amounts of weight since first appearing in public. I feel this would be an important article because, these magazines are criticizing the actresses for being too skinny, yet at the same time, putting them on the cover of their magazines so young women can dream of someday having their figure.

Seventeen

Draft 1

Megan Wells

While glancing at my sister's collection of magazines one afternoon, I was extremely disturbed at what I observed. Among the heap of random magazines, I spotted one of the more popular teen magazines, "Seventeen." I couldn't believe what they had picked out to be on the cover of their magazine, no wonder many teenage women have eating disorders. Patrice G. Adcroft, the editor of the ever popular magazine, "Seventeen" (2000), presents an all to familiar beautiful, young girl dressed in tight clothing with mounds of makeup piled on her face. The rest of the lay out of the magazine cover also possess "catchy" subtitles that are both inappropriate and sexist.

When I look at this magazine cover, I feel outraged. Why does the media insist on only putting the skinniest women they can find on the cover of their magazines. Don't they know that they are conveying a very bad massage to all those young women of the world? I guess I am also a little biased towards this situation because I have dealt with the issue of anorexia in my family for over a year now. Ever since my little sister has hit high school, she has been completely obsessed with her appearance. This has taken a great toll on both her and the rest of our family. I believe that these magazines she subscribes to are a big part of the problem. When you walk into my little sisters room, the first thing that you notice are the images on her walls, there hangs most of these hideous pictures from the front cover of Seventeen magazine. She defends them with pride if you try to question her taste in decorating.

Seventeen's May 2000 issue has a pink color theme to it. The focus of the text is obviously Rachael Leigh Cook, a young actress dressed in a provocative tight, little pink shirt. They positioned her so she is leaning to the right side of the cover and has one hand in her hair, and the other across her stomach pulling her skirt down, revealing a little skin. Her tank top is very fitted, especially across her chest. It is obvious that this shirt is made to accent the chest region. The shadowing in this shot also makes her chest look bigger because it is darker in the bottom half of the chest region as well. You can tell they want to make the shot a little more sexual, because of the way her hand is placed in her hair, as if she is being flirty with the cameraman. Her left hand is laid across her stomach just to the left of her pelvic area. Her right hand is also at a downward slope as if pointing to a certain region of the female body, as well as lowering her pink skirt showing her mid section ever so slightly. Again, I believe this is to show the more sexual side of this young girl.

Another interesting point of the cover is that, certain parts of the girl are covered in writing, while others are left untouched. The top of her head and her fore head area is covered with the title of the magazine, while the hand going to her hair is covered by a small subtitle. The heading of the name of the girl covers the right side of her body, the opposite side of where her left hand is placed. The only parts of this girl's body that aren't covered with any writing are her chest, and the part of her hand that is revealing her stomach. The cover definitely points you to what areas of the young girl they want you to observe.

On the left side of the cover, there are a few subtitles that are very sexual. One that is in bold letters at the top of the page reading, "THE BOYS OF BUFFY UNZIPPED," another reads, "How Far Would You Go For Him." This teenage magazine is just screaming SEX! No wonder kids today are more sexually active then ever before, look at what the media is putting out for them to read!

Personally, I think this text is geared for men. Every aspect of this cover is screaming sex. I don't see how women would find this appealing to look at. I think when young girls look at this magazine; it makes them feel that they need to look like the model in front of them. This is where their appeal for the magazine comes into play, their obsession of what society views as beautiful.

When comparing this text to other magazines, it is very similar to all other teen magazines. They all have the common theme of sexual appeal among young adults. As I talked about before, this has many possible affects on society. I think these magazines play a big role in teenage anorexia and bulimia, they help support the image that skinny is beautiful. Every new teen idol that comes out of Hollywood is placed on the cover of this magazine and ridiculed into another sexual object for women to worry about and men to dream about. The magazines also throw out the issue of teenage sexuality and backs up the controversial issue that teenage sex is okay. Perhaps the magazines popularity should be used to convey positive messages to young adults. It would be interesting to see what would happen if Seventeen suddenly started putting young women of normal or average weight on the cover of their magazines. I would guess that the younger generation would eventually become a lot healthier and happier about themselves, and life in general. Growing kids are under enough stress as it is going through the hormonal time in their life; this would be one less thing that they could stop worrying about.

Young and Modern

Draft 2

Megan Wells

"Young and Modern," with chief editor Diane Salvatore, is a magazine that used to be very familiar to me. During my earlier years in high school I used to be a monthly subscriber, but now as I observe the cover, I am appalled that this used to be part of my reading material. It has been so long since I have looked at this magazine, I laughed at the type of material they decided to publish in it. After analyzing the "Seventeen" magazine cover, I see many similarities between it and "YM."

Unlike "Seventeen" having just one young beautiful girl on the cover, "YM" has three. They are from the popular band, TLC. Looking at this text, the first thing I noticed was how skinny these girls were. What kind of message is this magazine portraying to young girls who are reading this material? Two of the girls have their stomachs showing, while the last on the left has a skin tight long dress on. I responded to this in such an aggressive manner because I know that once again, average, healthy women do not look like this, nor dress in this manner. I also feel ashamed that "YM" thinks it has to put this type of picture on its cover in order for the magazine to sell. I think this magazine is geared towards teenage girls, but why do they always put women on the cover, why not attractive guys?

This cover is arranged so that the three young women on the cover are the main focus. The background is white, which usually signifies purity. The woman on the left is wearing a velvet dress that is silver in the front and black on the back. Since the front of the dress is silver and form fitting, you can see all areas of her body. Her navel is especially apparent, along with her breasts. There is extra material that covers the groin part of her body, perhaps to draw more attention to it. At the same time it could mean that she is innocent, and that part of her body is something that she wants to keep hidden. She is also wearing pig tails in her hair to signify even less maturity. She is also wearing large silver hoop earrings, and a large silver ring on her middle finger that would represent her immaturity even more. As I have observed, most people who wear jewelry like this are a bit young and are still experimenting on what is cool to wear and what is not. Although she has all the signs of being an adolescent by the way she is dressed, a tattoo is very apparent on her arm. This is so large that it covers most of her upper arm, the tattoo says "Patton" with a stake going through a heart. The expression on her face is a bit odd. She looks as though she might be a bit scared of the camera, with those wide brown eyes. After examining her whole attire, I would conclude that she signifies innocents, and immaturity, yet at the same time has a bad girl side to her.

The girl in the middle, is wearing a grey sports bra with a grey leather looking dress. Her whole abdomen is showing which would represent the sexuality of a fully matured women. Her hair is tossed back from her forehead, and she wears a big smile on her face. Her smile is also seductive looking which could signify her wantingness for something.

The third women on the right, is wearing a rope shirt with a smaller tank top underneath it. You can not see her other clothing since most of her body is not shown on the page. Her hair is fire red and thrown back as though the wind picked a fight with her red locks. She is also wearing tiny diamond studded earrings that's telling the viewers that she is also a delicate type of woman. She is leaning over the women in the middle and looking straight at the camera. Her face is completely seductive looking, her eyes are slanted and mouth just barley in a smile. Her entire outfit and look on her face screams sex.

The three women's arms are entwined in one another as they are leaning in towards each other. This kind of touching and connection signifies togetherness, maybe even love for each other.

This text is totally set up so the main focus is on the three women. The only parts on the cover where there is no text, is on the women from their stomach areas, to their hair. The text in the cover also connects this picture from start to finish. You start by glancing up at the over sized purple letters, "YM," then work your way down the page reading the text which always ends on parts of the women's bodies. Then once you are finished, there is a caption about the singing group that is placed right below the women in the middle's stomach, which leads your eyes right to her exposed area. There is also a main theme with the text and the picture on the cover. Most of the text on the cover says stuff like, "How Guys Really Think," or "Could You Ask Him Out?" This is all stuff leading towards that sexual side of the reader, while the image of the three women screams seduction and sex itself!

I think the text is supposed to be geared towards younger women who are going through that maturing state. During this time, they are always wanting to talk about sex and their own bodies. Although, I think guys would get much more out of the cover then girls do. My impression is that girls look at this cover and envy the beautiful girls that are on it, while guys look at it and want to get with the women. I think the text is geared to be written from a teenagers perspective, but I still think they are being way to sexual with this age group. At that point of time in ones young life, you are very persuaded by anything that is put in front of you.

Basically, I think this cover coincides with the "Seventeen's" cover in which they scream sex. I think "YM" tries to portray it more innocently, but still manages to put their purpose out. They are portraying a message that sex and dressing sexy is alright, and the "right" way to show who you are. I think this type of text, helps make it okay for the other teen magazines to put this kind of stuff on their covers. As I said in my last essay, these magazines have a huge impact on teenagers and how they act. They are growing up around these magazines which kind of become their source for what is popular and what is not. This needs to be changed before every teenager tries to go through great lengths to look and act like these role models on the cover of magazines.

Teenage Idols

Draft 3

Megan Wells

In today's society, there is an increasing amount of pressure on teenage girls to have the "ideal" body. A big part of this pressure is due to what they are forced to face everyday on the cover of popular magazines that are geared towards their age level. Women that are picked to be on the cover of such magazines always look similar. These women are beautiful, full of make up, and excessively skinny. Because of this constant pressure to be "beautiful," teens go through great lengths to make themselves fit this persona, many times this means turning to Anorexia and bulemia. In this essay, I will talk about three different popular teen magazines, analyze what their covers look like and how they would effect growing adolescence.

After conversing with my younger, fifteen year old sister, I found out what some of the more popular teen magazines were. She gave me the names of *Mademoiselle, YM,* and *Seventeen*. Going out on a limb to prove my point, I trusted her opinion and bought all three magazines. What I found was appalling.

The first magazine that I analyzed, is the popular *Seventeen*. On the cover of this magazine, there is a young girl dressed in a cute pink outfit. Just glancing at the cover you would think that it presents itself as pretty innocent, but after analyzing it I became more disgusted. The theme of the cover is obviously pink since both the background and the girl are wearing pink. This theme is to signify the feminine part of the young girl. The shirt that Rachael Leigh Cook, the young actress is wearing is very provocative. The shirt is fitted, especially across her chest, you can tell this shirt was made to accent the chest region. The shadowing in this picture also enhances her chest making it bigger and more prominent. Rachael is also positioned so she is leaning to the right side of the cover, having one hand in her hair, and the other across her stomach pulling down some of her skirt. The significance of her hand pulling down part of her skirt to show some of her stomach is to show the more sexual side of the actress. The fact that her whole arm is laid across her pelvic area, just screams that this is a place in need for some attention. This could also symbolize the more sexual side of the actress. Her body structure again is extremely small. Because she is so skinny, her body makes her look young, so the magazine photographers had to cover this by slapping a bunch of make up on her face, and had her wear clothes that would accent the more sexual parts of the woman.

"YM," or also known as *Young and Modern* had a little different cover. This cover includes a picture of the popular singing group, TLC. The first thing I noticed about this text was how skinny all three girls were. Two of the girls have their stomachs showing, and the third has a skin tight velvet dress on that accentuates both her female parts and her skinniness. The background of the cover is white, this is to have the reader focus more on their bodies because they are black which stands out against a pale background. The woman on the left, Lisa, is wearing a velvet dress that is silver in the front and black on the back. Since the front of the dress is silver, you can see all the feminine parts of the body. Her navel is especially apparent, along with her breasts. There is also more material that covers the groin part of her body, perhaps to draw more attention to that this sexual area of the female. Lisa's hair is pulled back in pony tails to symbolize the more adolescent side of her, but at the same time she has a tattoo to show that bad girl side of her.

The woman in the middle, Tionne, is wearing a gray sports bra with a gray leather looking skirt. Her whole midriff is showing revealing her skinniness as well as representing the sexuality of a fully matured woman. She has a great seductive smile on her face signifying her wantingness for something.

The third woman on the right, Rozanda, is wearing a white rope shirt with a smaller tank top underneath it. The rope shirt comes across as extremely sexy because it leaves nothing to the imagination. This lack of clothing also shows her skin and bone body. The rope shirt could signify a net in which she is wrapped in, making her just an object of someone's find. Her seductive smile on her face tells the reader that she wants a little more then your attention.

The last magazine I analyzed was, "Mademoiselle." On the cover of this magazine is the famous Minnie Driver. The background is white which accentuates her tan, thin body. She is wearing a tiny purple string bikini top with a purple wrap around her hips. The way her tan is, there is a small white line that is between her breasts which points out this part of her body even more. Part of her breasts are not covered by this tiny bikini which makes this picture more sexual. The bikini is made so it sets her breasts very wide towards the sides of her body. This accentuates the largeness of her chest. Holding the bikini together, there is a silver metal clip in the center of her chest. Since this is such a color contrast to her skin tone, it draws your eyes into this area even more. Her whole abdomen is showing exposing her skinniness and firm body. There is absolutely no piece of fat on this woman's body, only muscle and skin. Her arms and hands are placed in a very obvious way. Her hands rest right on the front of her hips which connect and form a straight line to her pelvic area. This area of the woman's body is usually very private, yet her it is very exposed. The way her arms are curled towards this area and hands resting on this place, makes a path perfectly to this area of the female body. Minnie Driver is wearing many beaded bracelets on her left hand and tiny beaded earrings. This jewelry matches the color of the rest of the outfit making her whole appearance more appealing.

The top of her head is covered by the title of the magazine which kind of draws your attention off this part of the body. Since her face is kind of obstructed, it makes her body seem even more of an object, not of someone's actual body.

When teen's view these images on the cover of their magazines, the kind of text that is included with the pictures prevents them talking about their own bodies but more in relation to how men view them. The kind of text that is mixed with the cover pictures are, "How Guys Really Think," and, "Could You Ask Him Out?" These covers make the women seem more of an object rather then a real person. It is as if women are looking like this for the pleasure of what men think, not about how they can please themselves.

With growing pressure both from the media, and society, there is an ever-increasing amount of teens that succumb to pain to try to look like the "beautiful" women they see on the covers of their magazines. In a way, these magazines become role models for many young girls, they tell them what is popular, and what is acceptable to wear and to look like. If this is all these girls have to look at, how can they be taught that this is not the healthy look they should be pursuing. As for the extremely sexual side of the magazine themes, I think this is totally unacceptable. Today, kids are becoming more sexually active at a younger age then ever before. This is partly because of the articles they read about how to make "their man" happy, or how to steal their hearts. These articles never talk about how they can strengthen their own personal self and be their own person. It is only how they can improve themselves for the guys they have crushes on. Tell me, is this the way we should be teaching our kids how to go through their maturing stages of life?

Teen Pressure from the Media

Draft 4

Megan Wells

Anorexia is an increasingly growing problem among many teens across the country. Because of this mental and physical disease, many teens become victim to severe illness and even death. *Seventeen, YM,* and *Mademoiselle* are all examples of popular teen magazines that reinforce controversial issues in society. Such controversial issues are teenage sex, sexist images, and the appearance of Anorexia.

Anorexia is a disease that affects usually a young person's mind to the extent that they think they are over weight. Because one has the power to control their body weight, they starve themselves to the point that their bodies become skin and bones. Even though they look extremely ill, they think their new appearance is beautiful. This pressure to be thin comes from a variety of places. The most prominent place is most likely from society itself. Society today is in love with the "beautiful" supermodels in their size zero clothing while still standing at six feet tall. Women of this same stature appear on 99% of the country's popular magazine covers; among them are teen magazines.

Anorexia has become a big part of my family's life. My younger sister, Caitlin, has become victim to this terrible disease. In her ninth grade year, she went from a size eight to a size zero in three months. The desire to be thin and popular was something she wanted more then anything. Unfortunately she has paid dearly for this new body. Because she has starved herself of the many nutrients her young, growing body needs, she now has major problems with her hips, stomach, and feminine parts.

Since Caitlin is dealing with this serious disease personally, and also subscribes to many of these popular teen magazines, I decided to ask her a few questions about this issue. "When I look at the cover of the magazines I subscribe too, I see beautiful skinny women whose clothes are tightly fitted to their bodies," Caitlin replies with a sigh. Asking her why she thought these women where picked to be on the cover of these magazines, she replies, "They are obviously perfect if they are on the cover of a nation wide magazine." My sister also pointed out that when she and her peers look at these beautiful women, it makes them depressed about the way their own bodies look, and encourages them to stop eating. "Some of the models on the covers of these magazines aren't even pretty, you just have to be skinny to be noticed and picked to be on them. But, I think that if women who were of average weight were placed on the cover, the magazines wouldn't be as popular because they wouldn't be as attractive to look at. This is not the image most girls want to see because they want to imagine themselves as becoming beautiful like the women they are surrounded by in society."

To Caitlin, the skinnier you are, the more popular you will be, more guys will be attracted to you, and this ultimately means you will be happier with your life. "Looking at these women encouraged me to be skinny because you see them always looking so happy in the pictures. I thought that if I were that size, then maybe I could be happier about myself again." When I asked Caitlin how big of a percentage her magazines affected her decision to lose weight, she gave me a figure of about 50%. Although my sister is 5'4' and a mere 100 pounds, she still refuses to think of herself as anorexic. She is in a constant struggle to lose even more weight in time for summer. I just wish she would let me help her get better.

When analyzing each magazine cover, there were many common themes that I found to be included in all of them. The most predominant were the figures of all the women. In the magazine *Seventeen,* Rachael Leigh Cook is the model posing for the cover. She looks to be about twenty years of age, yet she has the bust of a mature adult woman and the body of a young child. The shadowing underneath her breasts increases their size, making them the main focus of the picture. Her left hand is placed around the front of her stomach, while pulling down a side of her skirt. This action made it possible to see her flat stomach and hipbone. The rest of her body is quite small and petite; the type of shirt she is wearing doesn't allow you to see her collarbone area, but her arms appear to be skin and bones.

YM has three women on the cover of their May 2000 issue. Lisa, Tionne, and Rozanda are from the popular band TLC. All three of these women are also very thin, but their breast sizes aren't apparent because of the way they are positioned in the picture. Since they are all standing sideways in the photo, you can easily see these women are very slender. Two of the women's stomachs are bare, and the type of lighting used to create shadows on their navel areas make them look even thinner. Their arms appear to be well toned, leaving no area for unwanted fat. On one of the women, her collarbone is in view, making it easy to see where her skin is sunken in around the upper part of her chest.

Minnie Driver, on the cover of *Mademoiselle*, leaves nothing to the imagination. Most of her body is in view due to the small bikini she is wearing. Although her body is petite, her abdomen is well toned and conditioned. Her breasts also seem rather large for the size of the rest of her body. Her skin seems flawless and tan. There is a substantial amount of shadowing that is apparent around the insides of her breasts, which make them more defined. The outside of her stomach area is also shadowed making her waist appear thinner. Her upper chest area is sunken in due to the lack of fat, making her collarbone and top ribs apparent.

Coloring and clothing can also have a great effect on how a particular picture is viewed. *Seventeen* has a color theme of pink in its May 2000 issue. Rachael Leigh Cook is wearing a rich pink tank top and skirt. The background of the photo is a slightly lighter pink. The color pink is usually the favorite color of young girls or infants. They could have used this color to signify the innocence of Rachael, or her youth. It is just puzzling to me that although they might want to portray her as a youthful looking woman, they choose to put her in clothing that is very provocative. Her tank top is so tight that it highlights the largeness of her breasts, while her skirt snuggly wraps around her hips.

The background color on the newest issue of *YM* is white. This is to make the three black women from the teen band TLC stand out more. Lisa, she is on the far left, is wearing a tight silver and black dress that helps to define her body. Since the back of her dress is black, her butt is very apparent while she stands sideways in the photo against the white background. The woman in the middle, Tionne, is wearing a gray sports bra with a gray leather skirt. Since her skin color is black, her stomach sticks out in this photo because of the color contrast to the background. The third woman, Rozanda, is wearing a tiny gray tank top with a rope shirt over it. The lower part of her body runs off the page, making it impossible to see what else she is wearing. The rope shirt could signify a net in which she is wrapped, making her just an object of someone's find.

Her outfit also stands out in the photo because of the gray vs. white contrast.

The background of *Mademoiselle* is also white. This color background makes Minnie Driver stand out well because of the darkness of her skin. She is wearing a small purple string bikini on top and a purple skirt on the bottom. The bikini really sticks out on her body because it is so dark on her lightly tanned skin. This also accentuates her chest because it is so tightly fitted. Holding the bikini top together is a small metal clip in the center of her chest. Since this is such a color contrast to her skin tone, it draws your eyes right into this area. Her skirt is also tightly woven around her hips, making her look even skinnier. Her hands resting on both sides of her skirt stand out due to the lightness of her hands and the darkness of the purple skirt.

The way a hand or arm is positioned on the body could have many different meanings. Rachael, in *Seventeen*, has her left arm wrapped around her stomach at an angle parallel to her groin area. This leads the viewer's eyes right to this private area of the female body. Her left hand is pulling down a small area of her skirt, revealing her stomach. Her right hand is in her hair; perhaps she is flirting with the viewer of the magazine. The positions of both her hands and arms signifies the invitation of sex.

The three women on the cover of *YM* have their arms entangled in one another, while their bodies are all facing each other in a sideways angle. This type of touching and body language could signify their closeness to each other, maybe even their love for each other.

Minnie Driver on the cover of *Mademoiselle* has her arms at a perfect angle, leading down towards the center of her groin area. Her hands rest on the front of her hips, while pointing ever so slightly inward. This area of the woman is usually very private, yet here it is very exposed. This could signify the sexual side of her.

The text along with the pictures on the covers of these popular magazines can be very persuasive towards being thin and dealing with sexual issues. On the cover of *Seventeen*, there are some headlines that include, "How Far Would You Go With Him," and "THE BOYS OF BUFFY UNZIPPED." On the cover of YM "Could You Go Out With Him?" and "100 Best Beauty Tips Ever." On the cover of Mademoiselle, "How Wild Does He Want It?" and "Celebrities Solve Your

Problems." All of these headlines are either dealing with issues about guys, or how to improve the way you look for them! What kind of message is this sending? These magazines show you pictures of beautiful, skinny women and then on the side tell you how you can be more like them. They are implying that these models should be your basis on what is beautiful. The text is also always talking about how to get a guy, or how to improve yourself to "score" one. This implies that they are pressuring you to be beautiful not for yourself but for the men out there waiting to be had.

With growing force both from the media and society to be thin, there is an ever increasing amount of teens that succumb to the pressure of Anorexia. In a way, these magazines become role models for many young girls. They tell them what is popular, and what is acceptable to wear and how they should look. If this is all these girls have to look at, how can they be taught that this is not the healthy look they should be pursuing. Today, kids are also becoming more sexually active at a younger age then ever before. This is partially because of the articles they read about how to make "their men" happy, or how to steal their hearts. These articles never talk about how they can strengthen their own self and be their own person. It is only how to improve themselves for the guys they want to impress. I think in order to improve these problems, society should take another look at what is happening to today's youth. My sister is a prime example of what can happen when young girls are pressured to be thin. Magazines that are geared towards teens should be more aware of how they present their material. Instead of skinny = thin and sex = relationships and fun, it should be more like fitness for better health, and no sex until you are more mature to handle the issue.

The Miseducation of Rap

Valarie Cook

Do you know what Gangsta rap is? Have you ever head of West Coast versus East Coast rap? If you heard old school rap, would you be able to tell it was old school rap from hard-core rap? Most people would answer, "no, I don't listen to rap." I probably would have said the same thing if I were not already tuned into the style of Eminem. When I say the word "rap" most people think of hard core beats, bad lyrics, and profane language. Not everybody realizes that some of these artists actually have something to say, and they can do it in very different ways.

The first style of rap is now called old school rap because it died in 1984. Old school rapping was easy to perform because it only required some microphones, a turntable, and somebody with good rhyming sense. This may surprise some people because the seventies, when rap was alive and well, is more commonly called the disco age, with later artists such as the Village People the Bee Gees, and Blondie all contributing to the beginning of rap. However, early rappers such as Run-DMC had less bass to their beat, and the raps always syncopated with the beats exactly. There was a lot less freestyle in the songs in comparison to today's rappers and this is why rap of today is said to be worse in terms of being productive and getting a point across.

Old school rap trickled into a completely new idea that received a lot of backlash due to their "hardcore" style. Hard-core rappers have the most difficult stereotype to break because of its intensity. Hardcore rap can be described as hip-hop that relies on driving beats. The sounds are always constant and in your face, and the lyrics are confrontational. Some famous hardcore rappers are Busta Rhymes, Master P, and Public Enemy. It is important to look past the stereotyped label of these artists to appreciate the value of their work. Not all hardcore rappers are out to spit as much as they can at the microphone and look like idiots. For example, Master P's song *The Master Plan* says "Teaches teens how to throw dice and pick locks. I wish you knew the issue. It's all wallet, politics. Done it, done it. Seen it, seen it. We seen it done." Although this phrase is surrounded by the image of harsh lyrics with harsh words from other rappers and other songs such as "nigga" and "bitches" this phrase is important because it is relating the artist back to something he knows and has seen. He is trying to address a real life issue about teens gambling and stealing, and he is able to do it in an effective way directly addressing teens about this issue. By acting as a vehicle of communication between generations, hardcore rappers are not just swearing and making money off of it. Instead they're finding ways to teach the next generation by speaking in terms of the world in which we live, not the censored world in which we are *supposed* to live.

West Coast versus East Coast rap sounds like a strange classification at first because the difference appears to be geographical, and not musical. The main difference between these two styles of rap is the record label from which they come. West Coast labels such as No Limit versus East Coast labels such as Universal International and Interscope chose the artists that will represent them based on the style of music the label is known for; regardless of the location from which the rapper comes. I still have a hard time differentiating the two styles, but I've heard that West Coast rap has a funkier beat, like reggae. The lyrics tend to focus on good times or fantasies. East Coast rap on the other hand is less funky, and is based more on what old school rap use to sound like. From these guidelines, a rapper from Maine can have a West Coast label as long as her style is funky just as a Californian rapper can have a record with an East Coast label as long as his beat is synchronized like old school rap. So the next time you hear somebody bashing West Coast versus East Coast rap you'll know that the difference relies on the record label and its certain style, and is not necessarily a reflection of Californians versus Bostonians. Alternative rap is a fairly recent and popular form of rap that has more of a West Coast feel, but draws from other styles of music such as funk, pop, rock, jazz, soul, reggae, and folk as well. One of my favorite alternative bands is the Fugees. Although their band has dispersed, their first big hit contained a great mix of different variations of alternative rap. For example, one of their most popular songs is called *No Woman, No Cry*. Sound familiar? Of course! This was one of Bob Marley's biggest and most popular hits. Bob Marley's style was certainly not ridiculed for profane language or harsh beats that were hard to follow, and thanks to the talent of the Fugees, this song was not massacred this way either.

Instead, they used a funkier beat to bring across the same mellow message as Marley himself; "In this great future we can't forget our past. So dry your tears, I say, oh, no women, no cry." Now does this sound like harsh hardcore rap to you? Is your perspective changing yet?

Last, but certainly not least, I would like to discuss a particular artist who has been singled out most recently for his harsh nonsense lyrics, confrontational attitude, and strange beats. Being white has also singled out Marshall Mathers because most rappers today are black, such as Dr. Dre, Jay-Z, Nas, Puff Daddy, and the late Notorious BIG. Most of the famous DJ's, spinners, and rappers are thought to be from ghettos of large cities, singing about things that only city people would understand. I believe that this is one reason why rap is usually not listened to in rural areas. When rap is not listened to, it can never be understood. I know that in my town, tiny Cabot, Vermont, you're considered strange if you listen to rap. You're viewed as one of the bad kids in school, and looked down upon by those who worship Britney Spears, N'SYNC, or any other flavor of the week.

Marshall Mathers, a.k.a. Eminem, doesn't consider himself to be any flavor of any week. With the release of every new record, Eminem has something to say about the response to his last record. As he claims, "you think I give a damn about a Grammy? Half you critics can't even stomach me let alone stand me . . . (*The Real Slim Shady*). The irony of Eminem's songs is that he sings to degrade people and then laughs about how he can get away with it. Many people who listen to this song find it offending and ignorant of Eminem to regard the Grammy award in this way. But they fail to see that the "Grammy" represents much more than the statue held up on stage. Eminem recognizes that he doesn't want to be seen as talented by the very people who have been discrediting him all year. He would rather have the attention from his fans. By using powerful words, and an image that makes you think twice about how truthful you really are, Eminem has become another misunderstood rapper in society's eye.

By expressing himself (when we know he's telling the truth) Eminem always manages to stir up controversy with his songs. However, does this one artist give a real perspective on how all rap artists express themselves? It certainly doesn't any more than a country fan could clump together Faith Hill's contemporary tunes with the whiny guitar of Randy Travis.

Music listeners of today need to learn how to interpret music independently of stereotypes. Rappers have mastered using beat instead of just words to express themselves, and this is why their words often seem harsh or profane out of context. So the next time you hear a rap song on the radio, don't change the station and dis the artist. Wait a few minutes and listen to what they have to say. You might relate to the pressures of life in general, even though you don't share the same lifestyle, and find yourself dancin' to the beat down the highway singing, "I'm so sick and tired of being admired . . . That I wish that I would just die or get fired . . . And drop from my label and stop with the fables . . . I'm not gonna be able to top what my name is" (*The Real Slim Shady.)*

Closer to Reality Than We Think

Kristin Williams

I am quiet and alone. I am sitting in front of my blaring computer screen with the lights off. The Olympics are on in the corner of my world, on my 10-inch TV screen, and I glance at it. A commercial flashes for Visa cards, somehow supposedly related to Olympic synchronized swimming. All of the ads on are trying to relate their product to the glory and athleticisms of the games. I stare off and then a commercial catches my eye. There is a view of a small house in the middle of the night, surrounded by woods. Then the camera goes into the house and a white woman with blonde hair is shown. Quiet and alone, much like me, she gets ready for a bath.

Slowly the camera shows her getting ready, she takes off her shirt, the camera follow it, and I see a cat at her feet behind her, who meows. America sees her white sports bra. She combs her hair sluggishly and opens her medicine cabinet. Putting the comb away, she closes it and in the mirror appears a guy in a white mask. The camera continues to move positions as the man lunges at her with a chainsaw and proceeds to chase her into the dark, daunting woods. I am confused. Why is an ad about some dumb horror film on at a time like this?

I am wrong, the commercial is not a movie promotion, it is a Nike ad. The commercial, I later learned, is called "Horror" and the woman is Suzy Hamilton, an Olympic athlete. In the end of the commercial I see the woman getting away, jumping over a log boundlessly, wearing a pair of running shoes. The masked murderer, who obviously didn't put on his pair of Nike's that day, puffs out of breath, and finally gives up. America sees, in small white case lettering, the question "why sport?" which Nike then answers for itself, "you'll live longer". By the end when I realize it is not an ad for a horror film but just another Nike commercial, I smile, I snicker, I huff, and then I feel enraged. I feel myself asking again why now? Why at all?

Why? The commercial was designed to produce an "edgy" ad that would make people look at sports in a new way (Nike in the News, Online). That is what Nike says. But truly, the point was to sell some shoes. And the ad got more attention than they ever expected it to get. People laughed and people were angry. The ad got so much attention that NBC pulled it off the air, and ESPN was not long to follow this action, because too many people were complaining. The vice president of US Marketing of Nike "We are disappointed . . . However this ad will continue to run in other media. Our rule has always been to respect the intelligence of our customer . . . we know they got the joke" (Nike Asks Sydney . . . Online). But apparently a lot of people didn't get the joke. They didn't get it as they sat down to watch the Olympics with their young children. I didn't get it as a female student sitting in my college dorm room alone. What I did get though, was that this ad was incredibly effective. Watching the advertisement closely one can observe a few reasons why. Nike uses the vulnerability of women right from the beginning. There are continually shots of running water throughout the beginning scene which build tension and create the idea that she is in a vulnerable state because she is about to take a bath. The viewer never thinks she is going to get away. She is blonde, a stereotypical attribute given to ditzy or stupid females. The emphasis on her white bra projects this image of innocence. The color white can imply this innocence; she is not, for example, wearing red or black. Also, it shows that she may not have any reason to wear a more sexual type of bra. We get this idea that this woman lives alone with her cat which is emphasized by this.

The use of sexuality of the woman is used as an attention getter, as is common in the media. When we first see her taking off her shirt there is this sexual nature about the ad. The running water, the focus on her blonde hair as she strokes it gently, the close ups of part of her face and the way the camera looks up her body after she has taken off her shirt all point to her sexuality. Furthermore, throughout the entire scene where she is being chased through the woods there is an emphasis on the upper half of her body. The viewer never knows what she is wearing other than her bra and her running shoes. The very dark setting makes the bra stand out even more. The advertisement also fooled the viewer, got them hooked and then twisted the ending to the viewers surprise when they discovered it was a Nike commercial. This ad was designed as a spoof off B horror films and was part of a series of "why sport" commercials, three total, that tried to look at "classic" cinematic moments in new ways. The problem with this ad that does not present itself in the other two ads of this genre that has the question "why sport" is that it takes a controversial issue fools the viewer and uses violence and sexuality to prove its point. The other two ads, "Elephant", where bicyclist Lance Armstrong saves a dying elephant by giving it mouth to mouth, and "Gladiator" where a skateboarder, in not much real danger, is followed by a gladiator, who smiles at the TV. (Nike Asks Sydney . . . Online)

Why then for the third ad did they turn to this? Nike, and many others, would argue that that in the same way that the other two are funny this one is too. As intelligent individuals we are supposed to be able to tell reality from fiction well. We know that the first two scenarios would never happen, it is fairly easy to get the joke. But do we really know about the third? Isn't half the enjoyment of watching a horror film the fear that it evokes? And what about the fact that the first two involve men where danger isn't present and the third about a female being attacked? And since when was coming after somebody with a chainsaw so funny anyway?

Well, apparently to many it is. Because the people who most likely thought that this ad was funny are the people who watch horror films with enjoyment. It makes sense that these people would laugh at the Nike commercial. The more one watches it, the less it becomes something to be scared of and the more it becomes something to laugh at. Suzy Hamilton said that she had wonderful feedback from teenagers and younger kids," and that her ten-year-old nephew loved it. (qtd. in Nike in the News, Online) This is the generation, myself included, who has been continually growing up exposed to greater amounts of violence on TV. These are the people who watch horror movies. Ten and getting the joke. Ten and laughing about a guy in a mask wielding a chainsaw and chasing a woman. What kind of message is that?

What is Nike really saying to its viewers? Well, maybe hey, if you buy our shoes they will save your life. Or, hey, if you are female then you should get out and do some running because you never know when you are going to need to get away from some man with a chainsaw. And hey, to that ten-year-old nephew, women being threatened with their lives are funny. Nike said themselves that the "'Why Sport' message expresses fundamental truths about sports in new ways" (Nike Asks Sydney.. Online). What is the fundamental truth they are getting at here? One might say that the ad in fact empowers woman and runners in general, but why should anyone be running?

The fundamental truth that Nike is projecting but isn't acknowledging is one America is seeing more and more of every time it turns on the TV. Let's look at MTV, look at Bay Watch, look at Jerry Springer. Look at video games. When I was younger I used to play Mario Brothers where cartoony short guys would walk around on different leveled blocks and the hardest part involved avoiding little fireballs. In the case in which he was hit, the man would just fall off the scene. Now there are all kinds of realistically rendered games where men and woman walk around with guns and shoot people and you see the blood spurting out of them as they die. And there are plenty of video games where scantly clad women with unrealistically large breasts fight other women like them. Is that empowerment?

Nike's ad caught a lot of attention because it was so racy. It succeeded, but at what cost? People make the argument that it is all about discerning the difference between reality and fiction. It seems as if parents, concerned about how well their kids can discern this difference, are the only ones complaining about the violence. I believe that you can't just blame TV for the lack of supervision that one gives their children. But I also believe that this effects everyone. Aren't we desensitizing ourselves to violence every time we watch it on TV? From insensitivity come acceptance, comes more violence. What we sit down and watch on TV reflects the way we choose to live as a society. The instant that commercial came on TV my reality changed; I was no longer just quiet and alone.

Their Eyes Were Watching God

Matthew Horowitz

> *Ships at a distance have every man's wish on board. For some they come in with the tide. For others they sail forever on the horizon, never out of sight, never landing until the watcher turns his eyes away in resignation, his dreams mocked to death by time. (1)*

In Zora Neale Hurston's *Their Eyes Were Watching God*, ships were on a collision course on the horizon, each one threatening to sink the others' dreams.

On the surface *Their Eyes Were Watching God* may seem like a simple story about a woman's life and marriages. However, the story is filled with conflict. As we follow Janie's life, her first conflict is with her grandmother. In Nanny's ship is the dream that her granddaughter will find security in marriage, so that she can die in peace. "Ah don't want yo' feathers always crumpled by folks throwin' up things in yo' face. And Ah can't die easy thinkin' maybe de menfolks white or black is makin' a spit cup outa you: Have some sympathy fuh me. Put me down easy, Janie, Ah'm a cracked plate." (20) Nanny was afraid that men would just use Janie without marrying her and giving her security and protection. Nanny is old and dying, but she cannot die in peace if someone else, a husband with 60 acres, is not watching out for Janie. Nanny's dream is in direct opposition to Janie's dream.

Janie had to hold back her own ship filled with her desires and dreams. She wanted to experience life and to fall in love, but her dreams and her grandmother's dreams were in conflict with one another. The two ships would collide if one of them did not retreat. So, Janie did as she was told and married an old man, Logan Killicks, in order for her grandmother's ship to come in. But Janie held out hope that love would follow marriage. "Finally out of Nanny's talk and her own conjectures she made a sort of comfort for herself. Yes, she would love Logan after they were married. She could see no way for it to come about, but Nanny and the old folks had said it, so it must be so. Husbands and wives always loved each other, and that was what marriage meant." (21)

The next ship to collide with Janie's ship was that of her first husband, Logan Killicks. In his ship was the dream of having a wife to do his work for him. After Logan and Janie were married six months, Logan started to tell Janie how his first wife did more of the work around the house. "Mah first wife never bothered me 'bout choppin' no wood nohow. She grab dat ax and sling chips lak uh man." (26) Janie was not going to chop wood and she told him that if he didn't chop wood, she wouldn't cook dinner. She might have won that battle, but soon after, Logan told Janie about his plans to buy a second mule so that she can help plow the fields. "'Ah aims tuh run two plows, and dis man Ah'm talkin' 'bout is got uh mule all gentled up so even uh women kin handle 'um.'" (27) Logan was no longer going to be the only provider in the family. He felt Nanny had spoiled Janie and from now on he expected her to work out in the field with him.

Love did not develop in Janie's first marriage, so she became restless. This time Janie's ship did not retreat. It sunk Logan's ship and she left him. This time she looked to the horizon through Joe Starks. "He spoke for change and chance." (29) Janie really thought her ship had come in this time. "From now until death she was going to have flower dust and springtime sprinkled over everything. A bee for her bloom. Her old thoughts were going to come in handy now . . . " (32) Janie thought she would finally find love with Joe Starks. Her thoughts returned to the days she spent under the pear tree dreaming of love and marriage. Her ship is sailing on the horizon again.

However, Janie is in for a rude awakening. Once again ships collide. This time Janie's ship retreated so far that if it had not been for Joe Starks' death, Janie's ship would have sailed forever on the horizon without ever landing. In her second marriage, Janie, once again, is treated like a possession. Only this time, instead of being a work mule, she is a trophy, a prized possession. Joe Starks gives Janie everything money can buy, but none of the emotional parts of marriage that Janie dreams of having. He does not let her mingle with the town or develop as her own person. "She had no more blossomy openings dusting pollen over her man, neither any glistening young fruit where the petals used to be. She found that she had a host of thoughts she had never expressed to him, and numerous emotions she had never let Jody know about. Things packed up and put away in parts of her heart where he could never find them." (72) Janie finally realizes that Jody will not fulfill her dreams. She has not found the love she dreamed of under the pear tree. She expected to share her thoughts and dreams with her husband, but Jody does not give her the opportunity to express herself and she knows he never will.

Joe Starks' ship carried a dream that he would be a "big voice." He wanted stature and all the status symbols of success. His dreams did not include allowing Janie to be herself because that would conflict with his ideas about proper behavior for the wife of a mayor. Joe Starks almost sinks Janie's ship. Throughout her marriage to Joe Starks, Janie loses sight of her ship and she almost drowns. When Joe Starks dies, her ship sets sail again. This time Janie is at the helm and enjoying every minute of it. "She was just basking in freedom for the most part without the need for thought . . . 'Tain't dat Ah worries over Joe's death, Pheoby. Ah jus' loves dis freedom.' 'Sh-sh-sh! Don't let nobody hear you say dat, Janie Folks will say you ain't sorry he's gone.' 'Let 'em say whut dey wants tuh, Pheoby. To my thinkin' mourning oughtn't tuh last no longer'n grief.'" (93) Janie is liberated by Jody's death. For the first time in her adult life, Janie can be herself, and sail her own ship on the horizon, rather than be the submissive wife of the mayor. She is through retreating or drifting on the horizon. Jody's ship is no longer blocking her path. Janie does not have to wear her hair pinned up under a rag. She can let her hair down. She does not want to pretend to mourn Jody's death when she is no longer sad about his death.

When Janie meets Tea Cake, their ships sail side by side. Janie finally finds love with Tea Cake even though everyone in Eatonville warns her against him. He is twelve years younger than Janie and a drifter. However, their two ships do not sail on forever. Tea Cake is foolish and he takes many chances in life. When a hurricane threatens the Everglades, Tea Cake ignores the warnings from the authorities to evacuate the Everglades. Janie and Tea Cake are caught in the storm. While trying to escape the rushing waters of Lake Okechobee, Janie is blown away by the wind when she picks up a piece of tar-paper roofing. She falls in the water and grabs on to the tail of a cow to keep herself from drowning, but she is almost attacked by a rabid dog who was riding on the cows back. Tea Cake saves her, but the dog bites him. When he develops rabies and attempts to kill Janie, she must shoot him in order to survive. Tea Cake's ship sinks and almost takes Janie's ship down with it. She is arrested for his murder and all of Tea Cake's friends turn against her. "They were all against her, she could see. So many were there against her that a light slap from each one of them would have beat her to death." (185) Tea Cake's friends are angry about his death and they want Janie to be their scapegoat. Blacks are not allowed to actually have a role in the white man's court so they must stand in the back of the courtroom without saying anything; however, their eyes are sending darts (or slaps) at Janie. They want Janie to be punished for Tea Cake's death.

Janie's ship did not sink. She was acquitted of Tea Cake's murder and his friends found a way to forgive her. When Janie returned home to Eatonville, she appears sad and tired. But we soon learn that her ship has come in. Janie is at peace with herself. She is no longer the submissive woman that gives in to everyone else's dreams. She is alone, but she has found herself. She no longer needs to sail on the horizon. "She pulled in her horizon like a great fish-net. Pulled it from around the waist of the world and draped it over her shoulder. So much of life in its meshes! She called in her soul to come and see." (193) Janie's ship collided with many ships in her life, but only hers reached the horizon. She now knows who she is and her dreams have been fulfilled.

To Tiffany & Co

Sarah Boucher

To Tiffany & Co. and the makers of Zippo,

Your ads deliberately target the fragile self-esteem of teenagers; you promote your products by promising the viewers lives of perfect romance and lots of money. You purposely cause your buyers to compare themselves to beautiful, rich Hollywood actors, and you cause your viewers to compare their lives to "Hollywood-style" lives filled with wealth. Your focus *should* be on the products themselves, not on these ideals that, for the majority of young adults, are nearly impossible to live by.

It is bad enough that there is a 24-hour service online that enables anyone to view the 450 foot long Hollywood sign as it appears at any time during the day. Maybe America should start using cameras for more constructive purposes; having a camera on the sign with 50 foot tall letters 24 hours a day just to remind average, middle-class Americans how "not special" they are is outrageous. Teenagers are influenced by Hollywood more than ever; according to a survey by Teen Research Unlimited of Northbrook, Illinois in 1997, of over 2000 teenagers polled across the nation, the majority of teenagers ages 13-19 "love" going to movies more than dating, shopping, and sleeping in. Janet Weeks, the author of a 1997 article for the Detroit News entitled "Hollywood Has a Growing Interest In More Teen Flicks," reported that this survey may also indicate that teen culture may dominate Hollywood film in the next few years. Teenagers spend more than $100 billion a year on clothes and shoes, pagers and cell phones, and movie tickets. Weeks believes that Hollywood has noticed this spending. Scream 2, a $24 million movie featuring teenagers, brought in $33 million; two-thirds of that audience was under 25 years old. David Davis, an entertainment analyst, said that Scream 2's success will prompt a major change in the economics of Hollywood. Hollywood once thought successful movies were those that targeted many age groups. In response to Scream 2's success, Davis responded, "I've been watching films appear weekly for nine years, and this is the biggest change I've seen. It's the first real shifting in the 1990s. The idea has always been that if you can make your movie appeal to the widest audience you can succeed. Perhaps that isn't so anymore. Maybe the new idea is that if you can succeed in targeting to your core demographic, you can make a good gross."

Aside from Hollywood films' influences on teenagers, your ads are attempting to take even more away from them: money and positive self-esteem. There is no doubt that your ads use Hollywood to promote two American ideals, wealth and romance, to target teenagers. The white Hollywood sign in the Zippo ad draws the eye of the viewer to its letters; simply the sign itself provokes teenagers' thoughts of money and a rich society of beautiful actors and actresses. The ad suggests that using Zippos can make one look more carefree and fashionable and live a life the same way—carefree and wealthy with an ideal member of the opposite sex. Like the tree in the Zippo ad, the rain in the diamond engagement ring ad is a life force; it is essential to life. Therefore like the Zippo, the engagement ring is necessary for a fulfilled live of romance and wealth. This ad looks like a scene from a romantic movie; the attractive young man and woman appear to be actors because of their flawless appearance, loving expressions and perfect stance. They also appear to be young because of their hairstyles, young faces, perfect complexions and the man's cleanly shaven face. The formation of their upper bodies is even in the shape of a heart—this would be considered a perfectly executed visual symbol for a film director. The city behind them is dulled because of the magic surrounding the couple and the headlights from the car appear to highlight the heavenly occasion—also a perfect, climatic scene for a romantic movie.

The romance element in the ad for Zippos is illustrated by the printed logo, "Use it to start something." This is a reference to a budding romance, which is appealing to teenagers who are beginning to learn about romantic relationships; they may even believe that using a Zippo will impress members of the opposite sex. The attractive couple on the page represents romance; the man and woman are young adults but their stylish, flowy clothes make them look like teenagers. The woman's legs are lit up and highlighted by the flame below, which may be the "fire" between the couple or the "spark" beneath them. She too is wearing a fun, flowy, outfit. Romance is prevalent because of the time in the ad—at dusk or early evening. This is shown by the sky and the way the purple fades from light to dark. The focal point of the ad is the deck underneath the couple, which is sexually suggestive, reinforced by the provocative smile on the woman's face. The scattered pots with flames and the flame beneath them symbolize heat and passion; sex certainly sells to teenagers. Purple is the prevailing color in this ad; according to J.L. Morton, adolescents or "the immature" prefer the color purple, therefore this ad is a clever target to young adults. Morton says that purple "is known as a magical, mystical bonding—a fusion of two into one. It is a blend of moderation and confidence." The fusion can refer to the couple itself, and teenagers are attracted to a sense of confidence that they may see in the couple, and therefore are attracted to the Zippo. The couple in the diamond engagement ring ad illustrates romance itself; an engagement is generally a romantic occasion. Aside from the romantically suggestive stance and stares of the couple, they are posed under one umbrella which unites the couple.

In the Zippo ad, wealth is illustrated by a fancy looking deck on which the couple is posed, overlooking what appears to be a pool. The pool, deck, and pots represent wealth, and certainly make it appealing to teenagers; anyone who owns a gorgeous pool overlooking the Hollywood sign would certainly have a lot of money; the setting also appears so beautiful and desirable because of the gorgeous hues of purple and shadows and reflections. Some teenagers associate purple with royalty; this may cause viewers to think of wealth when they see the color purple. The diamond engagement ring ad illustrates wealth through the design of the ad itself; the engagement ring is centered with its own shadow against a white background that takes up half the page. The raindrops falling from the umbrella look like diamonds. The clothing of the couple appears to be expensive; even the box uniting the couple's hands is held closed by a neatly tied white bow. And finally, in small print, the most prominent example of wealth in the ad—the price of the engagement ring. From $950 to $950,000.

Teenagers are exposed to Hollywood and its symbols nearly everyday; Hollywood has even changed their focus to hiring more teenage actors and actresses because the teenage audience has grown so drastically. It is very disturbing that you deliberately take advantage of teenagers and lower their self-esteem regarding their own lives to sell your products; it is also pretty sneaky of you to use the work Hollywood has already done to target teenagers to sell your products. In future ads for your products I hope to see less focus on idealistic wealth and romance and target adults who in most cases actually have the money to spend and who are generally less insecure and more knowledgeable about romance.

Thank you,

Sarah Boucher

Running in Circles

Courtney Bancroft

The text that I decided to analyze is a song by Tracy Chapman entitled "Fast Car." This song first aired in the early nineties and has been playing on the radios ever since. The song is about a person —most likely a girl— that has had a difficult past. She has endured many hardships and has grown up well beyond her years. The basis of the story is about how she wants to run away and start her life over. Towards the end of the song an irony is expressed that seems to send her life in a circle. The girl, now a woman, realizes that she is now living with exactly what she was trying to get away from.

At the beginning the girl in this song is old enough to realize that the time has come when she needs to live her life for herself. She was burdened at a young age with the responsibility of taking care of her drunk father and seems to have never truly experienced what it means to live—"I said somebody's got to take care of him so I quit school and that's what I did." She has taken on too many responsibilities at too young an age, and now all she wants to do is, "leave tonight or live and die this way." The irony in this statement is that she will, inevitably, die this way.

Towards the ending of the song we, as listeners, find that the woman's life has not significantly changed. She still has a man in her life that pays more attention to the bottle than he does to her. Also, living in a shelter does not seem that she has "Finally see(n) what it means to be living." The lyrics, "You stay out drinking late at the bar / See more of your friends than you do of your kids / I'd always hoped for better / Thought maybe together you and me would find it" show that she had always hoped for better, but now she has lost all hope and knows that she needs to get out. The words expressed here take me back to the part of the song where we learn how her mother left her father because he was a drunk—"My mama went off and left him /She wanted more from life than he could give." Her life has turned out to resemble that of her mother's life. Though we do not know her mother's past, we do know that she ran away because of the problems caused by her drunken husband. Now, the little girl that wanted to leave to be free of her burdens has grown up and is now enduring the same burdens that she was trying to get away from—a drunken man who does not have any respect for the women in his life.

The word choice in this text also helps to portray its deeper meaning In the beginning of the song words such as "together" and "we" are used many times. This shows how much emphasis is put on the girl and her boyfriend making a difference together. She is tired of people relying on her and, for the first time, she is depending on someone else to help her start a new life—her boyfriend. It seems that the girl has never had anyone that she felt secure around, so she is desperately trying to do so. The fifth verse says, "But it is fast enough so we can fly away / We gotta make a decision / We leave tonight or live and die this way." On the other hand, as the song continues to progress the words "together" and "we" are not used anymore. Chapman instead uses words like "you" and "I." This helps to show that the man and woman are now emotionally separated from each other.

In the last stanza, instead of focusing on togetherness, the word choice is suggesting that the girl is becoming more independent and has realized that the man she once wanted to run away with is now that same man that she wants to get away from. The last verse of the song states, "But it is fast enough so you can fly away / You gotta make a decision / You leave tonight or live and die this way." The woman seems to have excepted the fact that she needs to get out of the relationship that she once thought would help her. She ran away from a drunk, and she is now trying to do the same thing. Although, in this case, she wants him to leave and, for once, she is not the one running. The words shown here help to portray the changes in the woman's character. The once little girl with little self confidence is now a strong woman who has gained the courage to try and make it on her own. Though she is still in a shelter, she has rid herself of the person that has been dragging her down. Hopefully she will take this new freedom and make the best of it.

Though my life has not been anything like this I could understand it because, once in a while, everybody has had a time in their lives where they want to run away from their problems. It is a natural impulse. The woman's problems are more severe then mine could ever be, but I can still relate. This song has shown that running away from your problems does not necessarily make things better.

In this song we see the girl grow from a teenager to a young woman. Her problems seem to be whisked away by Mr. Wonderful who turns out not to be so wonderful. Ironically, he turns out to be just like the man she was trying to run away from—her father. This cycle is evident in our society and happens more often than it should. Women who have grown up in environments such as these tend to be prone to end up in the same situation as adults. The woman has ended up with a drunk for a husband and is in the same position as her mother was. Her life has made a complete circle, and she is finally mature enough to try to make it on her own. Finally the woman does not have to run anymore. She has found security and strength from her past experiences as well as other people's weaknesses, and hopefully she will use this strength to change her life around for the better.

The Sound of Silence

Bailey Gingras

'The Sound of Silence' is such a deep rooted and powerful song that it is often misinterpreted or not understood. It was written by Paul Simon, one of the greatest songwriters of a generation, in 1964, a time when the balance between hope and despair was in constant turmoil. The state of the nation was one of political and social upheaval with the war in Vietnam intensifying and rioting on the home front. But Simon never considered his songs political. "My strength is not political writing," he said in a 1984 interview with David Frieke, in New York's legendary songwriting factory, the Brill Building. "Those songs were about the mood of the times, but they weren't political." However, 'The Sound of Silence,' has not only strong relevance to that time, but to our own as well. It is a song about human nature, and that is a thing that may never change.

> Hello darkness, my old friend,
> I've come to talk with you again,
> Because a vision softly creeping,
> Left its seeds while I was sleeping,
> And the vision that was planted in my brain
> Still remains
> Within the sound of silence.

The song starts off slow with the first verse. Simon is talking to darkness, about a vision he had while he was sleeping. I find it interesting though, that the vision was planted in his brain, rather than in his mind or heart. Also, take note of how he uses the words 'softly creeping,' and how he refers to darkness as his old friend, meaning that Simon is an old acquaintance. He seems to imply that he has many times talked to darkness, and that it is a trusted confident Just the word darkness makes the listener think of evil-places to shy away from- and we wonder why this man could be his friend, and weather he himself is evil, or the darkness means something else all together.

In restless dreams I walked alone
Narrow streets of cobblestone,
'Neath the halo of a street lamp,
I turned my collar to the cold and damp
When my eyes were stabbed by the flash of a neon light
That split the night
And touched the sound of silence.

In the second verse the song rapidly gains speed. He describes having this incredible vision of a bright neon light splitting the night and touching the sound of silence. The phrase 'halo of a street lamp' puts us thinking that the vision came from God. I notice that he is walking alone, and that he receives this vision when he turns his collar to the cold and damp. The fact that the vision came to him through his eyes makes me think again about the seeds in his brain. Where is this bright neon light really coming from? He uses the word, stabbed, a violent intrusive word, like the contents of that vision were painful to him. I also find this verse in contrast to the first, when he refers to the vision as softly creeping. I think the contrast is there because he is expressing the way his unconscious feelings, which were elusive and creeping, very suddenly organized themselves into a striking and fearful realization.

And in the naked light I saw
Ten thousand people, maybe more.
People talking without speaking,
People hearing without listening,
People writing songs that voices never share
And no one dare
Disturb the sound of silence.

In the third verse he describes what he was shown in the vision. When he says, 'naked light,' he is emphasizing on the fact that what he saw is completely true and unprotected or disguised. He also talks about ten thousand people talking without speaking and hearing without listening. It is his way of saying that people no longer know how to speak their minds, or if they do, they dare not because they are afraid of disturbing the sound of silence. Silence is what is blocking the truth, the barrier between the restless emerging awareness within ourselves and an understanding which we are afraid to realize. Silence can't be heard, so the truth can't be heard, and people can't even begin to fathom its meaning. The ten thousand people can't even begin to break through because they lack the will to do so; they are not only not speaking, but they are not listening to the light in other peoples' voices. Simon puts in a glimmer of hope, then follows it with frustration. These people were writing songs, meaning that inside them there are great things being unearthed, but they lack the strength to share those songs with others for fear of disturbing the sound of silence. It is interesting how his voice sounds almost mournful when he says, 'and no one dare,' like not even one of those people has the courage to confront silence, or even try to approach it. Simon's tone suggests that that desire and awareness is what he craves for those people to understand. If they can not, do not dare to ask the question, how will they ever be able to search for the answer? He tries to help them.

> 'Fools' said I, 'you do not know
> Silence like a cancer grows.
> Hear my words that I might teach you,
> Take my arms that I might teach you.'
> But my words like silent raindrops fell,
> And echoed
> In the wells of silence.

I think the line 'silence like a cancer grows,' is a very powerful statement. To me cancer is a vicious disease that kills thousands; it is very painful, unstoppable, and uncontrollable. He is comparing it, a very real and tangible disease, with the idea of silence, the barricade that stands between the people in his vision and God and the truth. He had a vision from God that told him of the disease of silence which is infecting and growing and spreading. He calls out to the people to hear him, not just to listen, so that he may take their arms and enlighten them before it is too late. But his words fell on deaf ears. Silent raindrops that no one can hear, that only echo in the wells of silence. The word wells makes me think of a deep hole, an abyss to fall into and never get out of. It also brings to mind a store, a never ending supply, like water from a well. Silence is a formidable and well established opponent against which Simon has no weapon.

And the people bowed and prayed
To the neon God they made.
And the sign flashed out its warning,
In the words that it was forming.
And the sign said,
"The words of the prophets are written on the subway walls
And tenement halls"
And whisper'd in the sounds of silence.

The first two lines of this verse are especially significant because God is again brought into the song. Not just God, but "the neon God they made." Simon is saying that the people created their own god, and he's bright and neon like they would want him to be. The word neon also brings to mind images like cheep beer, bars, and strip joints, which brings up the question of what kind of God it is we have made for ourselves. Remember he had the vision when he turned his collar to the cold and damp, looking into the places where most people look away. He had the courage to search for the truth and also the wisdom to make sense of it. But the sign that the peoples' God gives them is far from neon; it says the very people who are deemed evil, or corrupt, who live on the fringes of society, and at times sanity, are the prophets themselves. Outcasts who scribble 'fuck you,' and 'the end is near,' and graffiti directions to the nearest drug house. But the people do not listen to what is spread before their eyes; their vision is blocked by the barricade of silence which is never broken. The answer to these peoples' prayers is whispered in the sounds of silence. But even Simon, who received a vision from God, can not teach them, can not reach them. I also find it interesting how in the last line of the first three verses the word sound is singular, but in the last verse, it is plural. This brings to mind the image of the seed and the cancer growing out of control. Even through the course of the song when he is calling out his warning, and the people are given a sign of warning from their own God, the sound of silence still keeps growing and spreading.

I think 'The Sound of Silence' is Simon's crown achievement as a songwriter. It is perfectly written, not a single word is out of place or without meaning. But beyond that it carries a message that transcends the barrier of time and expresses a warning about what he sees in society that is smothering true being. Even though this song came out of a time when the country was in upheaval, I don't believe we have yet solved this problem or even begun to face it.

White Expectations

Steven Pettrone

It is only possible to dream of a world where everyone can be who he or she was meant to be. We can only dream of a time where physical appearance means nothing, where the blind man sees just as much as a man with sight. We can only dream of a time and place in society where people of color don't have to placate to the white man's rules and the white man's expectations, a place where the color of a man's skin has no baring on his social status. *The Bluest Eye* by Toni Morrison is a novel that depicts the racial barriers in American society, and how the darkness of a person's skin can either create or shatter their happiness and stability.

In the first chapter of the novel, Autumn, the narrator, Claudia MacTeer, tries to explain the difference between being "put out," and being "put outdoors" (17). In this explanation of being removed from one's home, Claudia also makes a statement about being a minority in a white society:

> "Being a minority in both caste and class, we moved about anyway on the hem of life, struggling to consolidate our weaknesses and hang on, or to creep singly up into the major folds of the garment. Our peripheral existence, however, was something we had learned to deal with—probably because it was abstract."(17)

More than just addressing being kicked out of a home, this is a statement that describes life's difficulties when you are a minority. Morrison uses the image of a garment to symbolize society. The minorities are symbolized by the hem of the garment, always on the outside looking in. It is as though they will never be a part of the garment itself, just a minute detail that is easily torn.

Claudia is an example of a minority who is on the outskirts of society, always looking in at how wonderful the lives of the more fortunate children are. In Winter, Claudia reflects upon the people who come from such towns as Aiken, Marietta, Mobile, and Newport News: "They go to land-grant colleges, normal schools, and learn how to do the white man's work"(83). This quote describes the race barriers based on how dark a shade of black the skin was. The lighter skinned children are deemed more acceptable in society. Their parents have better jobs, and the children can go to high-class, white schools. At these well-endowed institutions, the lighter skinned black children learn how to be white. When these black children learn how to be white, they lose a sense of their native heritage, and also a sense of self. These black children have been given the opportunity to succeed in the white man's world; they pay to be taught how to be someone who they are not. This is an example of how higher society favors those who have lighter skin tones.

The training of becoming whiter consists of getting rid of the funkiness: "The dreadful funkiness of passion, the funkiness of nature, the funkiness of the wide range of human emotions . . . they fight it and fight it until it dies"(83). The children of towns like Aiken go to school to learn how not to be black. They are taught to mask their emotions for nature, passion, and blackness. Since lightening their skin color isn't feasible, they change their personality instead. They are taught to behave like white people and show no signs of their African heritage because it will only diminish their chances of success in the white dominated world.

Maureen Peal was a character who had lighter skin than most, which helped her acceptability within the white society.

> "Black boys didn't trip her in the halls; white boys didn't stone her, white girls didn't suck their teeth when she was assigned to be their work partners; black girls stepped aside when she wanted to use the sink in the girls' toilet, and their eyes genuflected under sliding lids."(62)

Though she has beautiful looks, Maureen has ugliness on the inside. She wasn't black like everyone else, but she did have darker skin than that of the white children. She was considered beautiful partly because she had lighter skin than her black classmates. Whether they were black or white, nobody would poke fun at her. In fact everyone looked up to her beauty. Who wouldn't be happy when everybody else is getting the hassle? Maureen is an example of how lighter skinned children were treated better. She is also an example of someone whose stability folds under circumstances that reveal her true heritage.

This buckling stability can be seen when there was a fight between Maureen and Claudia, over who was black and who was not. Maureen screams, "I am cute! And you ugly! Black and ugly black e mos. I am cute!"(Pg. 73) Maureen has made a life-long attempt get rid of the funkiness. She doesn't want to believe that she has African roots because such a background would make people look at her as if she was inferior to the white society that she dreams of being a part of. She has conformed to the white man's society so that her life would be made easier. Because she has beauty, the kids at school don't believe that she has any black inside of her. This creates a false sense of stability for Maureen.

Another example of a white person in a black body is Geraldine. Geraldine has a problem with the dirty black folks who she calls "niggers." She herself is black, but does not want to believe it. She will only allow her child, Junior, to play with white and colored people, not "niggers": "They were easily identifiable. Colored people were neat and quiet; niggers were dirty and loud. He belonged to the former group"(87). Junior always had a deep yearning to play with the black boys, because what he found to be fun in the black boys was their toughness, and reality of their presence, which he did not find in the white children. His mother would not approve of such play because she is afraid that he will not conform to the white man's ways and means. Interacting with other black children would, according to his mother, weaken the chances of Junior making a presence in the world.

As you can see, *The Bluest Eye* is full of examples of people desperately seeking to become a part of the white society, because of material benefits. Such greed and conformity leads to a loss of roots and heritage. The characters that choose to conform to the white man's ways truly believe that they are ugly, and that the only way to rid them of this ugliness is to walk, talk, think, and eat like the white man.

Research-Based Writing

Portfolio Introduction

Lauren Brown

I wrote many research papers throughout high school, but this assignment approached research in a different way. For this assignment we had to write an annotated bibliography, something I had never done before, a feature style draft, conduct an interview, complete an I-search, and write a final paper in magazine article format. This process was different and new to any other research paper I had written before. I decided to write this paper on something that meant a lot to me, my religion, Wicca.

Writing an annotated bibliography helped to start the assignment off. By looking through a variety of sources I was able to figure out more of a direction that I wanted to take my final draft in. It also helped with the general research of the paper because if I was looking for a specific item to include in my paper I could refer back to my bibliography.

The second draft helped me to see what direction I did not want to take my paper. Although my draft followed the assignment I did not see it as interesting, just informative. This draft helped because it allowed me to try one approach to my paper.

My third draft was my interview. Although I did not use this in my final draft it definitely helped get me on the right track. After I did my interview I knew that I wanted to focus on the discrimination against Witches and Wiccans in the US. I sort of got the idea too that I wanted to look at the topic from a personal view.

The I-search draft did not really contribute that much to my final draft but it was useful to learn how to do one. I have never had to write out my process before and I can see how by leaning how to write it out, I could have taken a different perspective on my final draft.

My final draft was my magazine style format. This draft was completely different from my other drafts. In this draft I took a completely personal look at my experiences dealing with discrimination. This draft is still a research paper though because information and research was included in the sidebars and within my article.

Draft Zero: Brainstorming

Lauren Brown

List five things over $100 you might possibly buy in the next year

1. TV
2. A nice dress
3. Winter Boots
4. A new CD player
5. textbooks

What do you spend your free time doing?

1. Reading
2. Answering E-mail
3. The Vermont Pagans
4. Drawing
5. Listening to music

What are the top three jobs you'd want (part-time while in school?)

1. Working for the College of Education (making web pages).
2. A bookstore (urn . . . free books!)
3. Something with children (daycare or something because it would help my career.)

Where would you most like to travel to &why?

1. Israel (I want to teach there someday)
2. Tahiti (I have always wanted to go there)
3. India (To experience the culture)

What are the three things you are most passionate about?

1. My religion (Wicca)
2. Art (drawing, painting, sculpting)
3. Piano

What are three things you've always wanted to learn how to do?

1. Paint nails
2. Dog grooming
3. Dance

If you were to open your own business, what would it be?
It would be a pet store that just sold turtles.

You've got three days to live . . . what will you spend your time doing?
Spending time with my family, friends, and pets.

What's the best way to spend a day off?
Sleeping.

If you had to teach a class, name three options.
1. Any elementary education class.
2. A class on the proper care of turtles
3. A computer class for little kids

What are three things you like about Burlington (e.g. vegetarian restaurants, lots of dogs, street performers)?
1. DOGS!!!!
2. All the little kids
3. The local artist shops

I would like to do something with my religion, Wicca. I think that I would like to do something along the lines of educating people about Wicca, and its beliefs. I could also do something on the resources for Wiccans in the Burlington community (shops, groups, the UVM group the Vermont Pagans). This topic would keep my interest for the whole five week with no problems at all.

Annotated Bibliography

Lauren Brown

Adler, Margot. *Drawing Down The Moon*. Boston: Beacon Press, 1986.

This book is an in-depth look at "Witches, Druids, Goddess-worshippers, and other Pagans in America today." It contains an interview done with a Wiccan High Priestess, and general information on the religion in the USA. It also includes history of Wicca and other pagan religions and some theories for why people are drawn to the religion.

This source will be extremely helpful because of the amount of history on the subject. I intend to give a brief history of Wicca in my paper. In this book Adler discusses many theories about how the Wiccan religion came about, this will be helpful because she also discusses why people are drawn to the Craft, a main point in my paper.

Boden, Audra. Personal interview. TBA.

Audra Boden is a student at UVM who has an interest in Wicca. Although she does not wish to become Wiccan at the time she is interested in learning about the religion.

Interviewing Audra will be helpful because although she has heard about the Wiccan religion she does not have any information about it. This will be a good source because Audra represents the average American, who does not really know anything about the religion except for what she has heard on TV or in the movies.

1) Where did you hear about Wicca?

2) Why are you interested in learning more about the Wiccan religion?

3) What do you think Wicca is?

4) Do you know any Wiccans?

5) Would you ever consider becoming Wiccan? Why?

Campbell, Andrew. "Vocal." *Vermont Open Circle Awareness League*. 23 June. 2000. Vermont Open Circle. 11 Nov. 2000. <http://opencircle.faithweb.com/VOCAU>.

This site contains information not only about the Vermont Open Circle, a coven located in the Burlington area, but about

Wiccans being vocal about their religion to help educate the public. "We are working to educate your community on the truth about Pagan religions—especially Witchcraft and other oppressed faiths. Through education, we can dispel the misconceptions that lead to ignorance and fear."

I will be able to use this site in two ways. One, it will give me a resource for Wiccans in the Burlington area for people who are thinking about becoming or finding out more about Wicca. Two, it will give some reasons that Wiccans that are in the "broom closet" should come out and be vocal about their religion.

Cunningham, Scott. *Living Wicca*. St. Paul: Llewellyn Publications, 1995.

Living Wicca is the sequel to Cunningham's *Wicca A Guide For The Solitary Practitioner*. This book has little information on actual practice of the religion, but contains a lot of information on the main concepts of the religion as well as information on designing your own traditions, telling people you are Wiccan, and teaching others about the Craft.

This book will provide good examples of the pros and cons of "coming out." It also has information on daily practice and a little bit about the history of Wicca, which can be used as additional resources for my paper. This book is also an excellent source to use because it is one of the most popular books to purchase for people new to the Craft. It will show the basic ideas that these people are learning.

Dunn, Mike. "Vermont Pagans Home." *Vermont Pagans*. 2000. University of Vermont 4 Nov. 2000. <http://www.uvm.edu/~vtpagans/home.html>.

This site contains information on a resource for Wiccans and Pagans on the UVM campus. There is information on joining the group, coming to meetings, plus the mission statement and constitution for the group. This site is currently under revision so some of the areas are not available to the public.

This site will be helpful because it provides a resource for Pagans and Wiccans at UVM. Because I am writing my paper about this subject (resources for people interested in Wicca) this site will be a good place to refer people to.

Kiziltan, Hale. Personal interview. TBA.

Hale Kiziltan is a UVM student interested in becoming Wiccan or at least looking into the religion in-depth. She was raised in a Muslim household which later converted to Christianity. She is exploring different religions currently to decide which one is right for her. Her information on Wicca has come from the media, books, and a few brief lessons from a Wiccan Priestess.

Hale will be an interesting and good source to interview because her background is typical of people who convert to Wicca (mixed religious training with some confusion). She has some knowledge of the religion so is not biased or ignorant about it. She has also had little contact with the Wiccan community in the Burlington area but would like too, this is the audience that I am trying to reach.

1) How long have you been interested in Wicca?

2) Have you practiced any Wiccan ceremonies?

3) Would you be interested in continuing your Wiccan education in a group setting?

4) Do you want to meet other Wiccans at UVM?

5) How did you hear about the Wiccan religion?

RavenWolf, Silver. *To Ride A Silver Broomstick*. St. Paul: Llewellyn Publications, 1997.

To Ride a Silver Broomstick ("New Generation Witchcraft") is probably the most common book for people to purchase who have just entered the Craft. It contains information on general history of the Craft, practice, and a large section about "coming out" and "challenging the shadows" (being vocal about your religion).

Although many Wiccans dislike Silver RavenWolf (due to the fact that she is trying to popularize the religion), this book will be helpful in many ways. It's section on 'To Tell or Not to Tell, That is the Question,' offers good advice on dealing with telling people that you are Wiccan. It gives the pros and cons of "coming out" including information about living in the broom closet ("There is nothing wrong with this as long as you are completely comfortable with it," and coming out "Once you have become comfortable with your beliefs in Witchcraft, you should sit back and consider how strong your personal convictions are.") This book will provide excellent arguments for both sides of the issue.

"The Craft Main Page." *The Craft*. 1996. Columbia Pictures. 2 Nov. 2000. <http://www.spe.sony.com/movies/thecraftl>.

This web site contains information on the popular movie *The Craft*. This site contains information on the making of the movie, the makers of the movie, the movie itself and information on a representative from Covenant of the Goddess, a Wiccan organization, who consulted on the film. "Pat Devin (Wiccan, or as she likes to call herself "Goddess in Residence") got into paganism at the age of ten but didn't start to identify herself as a 'witch' until around 1966, when Donovan recorded *Season of the Witch* . . ."

This site will help me because it will give me information on a popular reason people become interested in the Wiccan religion, media. By looking at this site I will be able to see how the movie *The Craft* appealed to teenagers and how it used Wiccan beliefs in the plot (even if incorrectly).

"The Witches' Voice: A News & Education Network." *The Witches' Voice*. Feb. 1997. The Witches' Voice Inc. 6 Nov. 2000. <http://www.witchvox.com/wvoxhome.html>.

This web page has information on just about anything anyone would want to know about Wicca. It contains information on current events and links to sites on general information, area sites (to locate Wiccans in your area), specialty sites, legal sites, and many others. This page is one of the most well known sources on the web, and is reliable.

This site will not only be helpful for finding sources in the Burlington area, but it will also provide general information on the topic, links to other sites (including those of people who have just "come out"), and just about anything else that I will need to find out or know about my topic.

"Vermont Wiccan & Pagan Resources." *Covenant of UU Pagans*. 15 Sept. 2000. First Unitarian Universalist Society of Burlington. 2 Nov. 2000. <http://hometown.aol.com/Firebearer/index. html>.

This is the official site of the Covenant of UU Pagans, one of the largest groups of Wiccans/Pagans in the Burlington area. It provides information about meeting times, contact people, about the group (mission, purpose . . .), and ways to get involved with the Pagan community in the Burlington area.

This site will also be a good place to refer people to in my paper who are interested in finding out more about the Wicca. It also provides links to other major Wiccan groups in the area, so that will also be helpful. This site is not as much of a research site as it is a place to refer people to.

Are You a Witch?

Lauren Brown

Are you a witch? Have you ever wanted to be one? Do you want to learn about real witches? I am not talking about the stereotypical witch, a woman with green skin and warts who flies around on a broom and eats little children on Halloween. No, I am talking about real witches, those who practice the religion Wicca, sometimes known as Wicce, the Craft, or Witchcraft. Real witches are walking around on your campus ***right now!*** Yet, what exactly is Witchcraft? How do you become a Witch? How do you find Witches if you are one?

Wicca, or Witchcraft is a Pagan religion that has roots dating back to before the start of Christianity. Pagan, originally being a term that meant "country dweller" in ancient Rome (Adler 9), is now used to describe a person that practices a religion that is not Christian, Jewish, Islamic, or considered mainstream. The word Wicca originally meant "to bend or turn." in Old English (Adler 10) This term was often used to describe midwives, herbalists, and early doctors. Wicca is now used to describe one of the fastest growing religions in the world. Scott Cunningham describes Wicca as "a loosely organized Pagan religion centering toward reverence for the creative forces of nature, usually symbolized by a Goddess and a God." The Wiccan religion almost died out during the Witch hunts a few hundred years ago, but made a comeback in the 1960's when Gerald Gardner informed the public that Wicca still existed. Wicca is now a religion that is recognized by the US government as a legitimate religion (in the armed forces and tax exemptions), and has somewhere between 50,000 and 200,000 members in the United States (the true number can not be known because many Wiccans are not public about their religion (Covenant of the Goddess).

The most important thing to know about Wicca is that it is full of variation. Every Coven, or group of Wiccans, or solitary Wiccan creates their own Book of Shadows, a book like the Bible. These books contain rituals, spells, and other important religious items. Although there is a lot of variation in the religion, all Wiccans have a few basic beliefs. Wicca is a nature based religion that celebrates its holidays on events in nature, such as solstices and full moons. Most Wiccans believe in a

Goddess and a God (often represented by the sun and the moon), but some just believe in one higher power that contains both sexes. Wiccans do practice magick (the "k" is to distinguish it from parlor tricks), which is similar to prayer. Wiccans do not (are not supposed to) try to convert anyone. Wiccans live by the rule "for everything that you do it will come threefold back to you." Many times if you are listening to Wiccans talk about their religion you will hear the phrase "And ye harm none, do what ye will." This comes from a poem called the Wiccan Rede, a basic summary of the Wiccan religion. Wiccans follow the Wiccan Rede, a poem by an unknown author that summarizes Wiccan beliefs. There are many branches of Wicca. A few main branches are: the "Old Religion," based on one's culture or heritage, Gardner Wicca or Traditional Wicca, based on the practices of Gerald Gardner; Dianic Wicca, a feminist form of Wicca; and Eclectic Wicca, the largest group of Wiccans who take many traditions to create a personal belief system. There are many other types of Wicca but many of them are similar to the types listed above.

If you are considering finding out more about Wicca, becoming Wiccan, or even learning how to cast a spell or practice magick there are lots of resources at UVM and in the Burlington community that can help you. The Vermont Pagans are one group on campus that is devoted to making the UVM community open to Pagans. Their mission is "to provide a safe, open, space for Pagans and the Pagan lifestyle. We exist to be active in both the University of Vermont community and the Burlington spiritual community." Not all the people in the Vermont Pagans are Wiccan, but they hold discussion meetings about once every other week to discuss different aspects of Pagan religions, including Wicca. The Vermont Pagans also plan workshops for people to learn about simple rituals in Wicca, such as casting a circle (a sacred space used by Wiccans before casting a spell). Because the Vermont Pagans are not all Wiccans they offer contacts to Wiccans on campus as well as groups off of campus. One major group of Wiccans are the Burlington Covenant of Unitarian Universalist Pagans. "The purpose of the Burlington UU Circle CUUPS chapter is to provide a safe place for Pagans in Vermont to create community and to assure through our ritual and other outreach projects that no Green Mountain Pagan is solitary unless they choose to be. Our most important services are providing a place for spiritual community, regular Pagan practice, and finding learning resources." CUUPS is a good place to go if you know nothing about Wicca. They have open circles (rituals that are open to the public) that anyone can attend. They will also put you into contact with other members of the pagan community.

If you are Wiccan or considering finding out about Wicca there are some things that you should take into consideration before you go and tell all of your friends and family. Although Wicca is a religion recognized by the U.S. Government there is still a lot of discrimination against it. At Fort Hood, in Texas, there is a large group of practicing Wiccans. Recently there was a large act of vandalism against them, estimated at over $3,000. A teacher in North Carolina was recently recommended to leave her job, which she did, because she appeared on a Wiccan web site. In Columbus, Ohio a girl was recently severely beaten by her father for owning books about Wicca. A girl in high school in Oklahoma was recently accused by her principle for putting a hex on a teacher and making him sick because she is Wiccan. And Presidential candidate George W. Bush was recently quoted saying "Whether Mormon, Methodist, Jewish, or Muslim, Americans should be able to participate in their constitutional free exercise of religion. I do not think witchcraft is a religion, and I do not think it is in any way appropriate for the U.S. military to promote it." Telling people that you are Wiccan or are thinking about becoming Wiccan is a major decision that needs to be made by each individual. When you are considering telling people that you are Wiccan make sure that you have knowledge about the basic practices and beliefs. You will be asked all sorts of questions ranging from "Do you believe in Satan?" (No, Satan is not part of our belief system), to "Can you put a hex on my ex?" (No, Wiccans are not allowed to hurt anyone). Make sure that you can defend the religion and that you can refer people to sources, such as www.witchesvox.com, for information. Also, remember that when you tell people you are Wiccan it means that you are locked into the religion, so make sure that you really want to be Wiccan.

Witches are real. They practice magick and cast spells. They live at UVM and you probably have met one. Wicca is one of the fastest growing but misunderstood religions in the country. If you are interested in leaning about Wicca, or learning anything connected with it contact the Vermont Pagans or CUUPS.

Interview

Lauren Brown

This interview with Audrey B (name has been changed) was conducted on 11/18/00 5:00pm. Audrey and I met in the lobby of our dorms to have this interview. The setting was relaxed and informal.

1) What is your religious upbringing?
I was raised strict Roman Catholic
Both parents?
Yes. When my dad was younger he wanted to be a priest.

2) What religion are you?
Roman Catholic. When I was home I went to church every week, now I go when ever possible.

3) What do you think defines religion?
I know this one from school (Audrey went to a Catholic high school). Religion is having a faith in God and looking for guidance from him in times of trouble in the form of prayer.

4) Do you believe witches exist?
No, absolutely not.

5) What do you know about witches?
Witches don't believe in God. They worship the Devil and they don't believe or care about heaven.

6) Do you think Wicca or Witchcraft is a religion? Why?
Wicca is not a religion. It was made up by pagans.
What is a Pagan?
Someone who does not believe in God. Beliefs that are man made not God made.

7) Where does your information on Wicca come from?
The movie The Craft and other movies. The book the Crucible. Hearing things about Salem Mass. Mostly the media though.

8) What is your opinion of people who practice Wicca?

They are out casts. They don't want to conform to Christianity so they make up own religion.

9) Have you heard anything about the discrimination/violence against Wiccans? If yes what and where did you hear it?

Yes, I heard about the persecution of Witches in History, like the Witch tests.

Anything recent?

No.

10) Have you ever known a Wiccan? If yes, what did you think of that about that person and their religion? If no, would you ever become friends' with a person who says they are Wiccan or a witch?

Yes, there was one who lived down the street for me. I felt that she did not have faith. I kind of pitied her.

11) Have you ever had any interest in Wicca as a possible religion, magick, casting spells, or witches in general?

Yes, as entertainment only though. I have never actually tried though.

12) What do you think Exodus 22:18 is saying: "Thou shalt not suffer a sorceress to live"?

First of all I don't think it is my place to interpret the Bible. You should ask a priest about that.

Can you give me an unofficial, personal interpretation of the passage?

Witches should not exist and if they do they should die? But I don't think that means that you should be killed or anything, I don't know. I don't think I can answer this question.

13) Do you think that Wiccans deserve the same legal rights as Christians (right to perform marriages, tax exemptions, practicing openly in the military)? Why?

No. They are not practicing a real religion, so they should not have religious freedom or any of those things. They are not on the same level as us [Christians].

14) Did you know that most/many Christian traditions came out of Paganism? What do you know about this? How does this make you feel about Christianity?

I did not know that.

(Explanation of history of the link between Christian and Pagan holidays.)

Ok, so our holidays were placed on the same day as yours. But ours are still right. I don't agree with the persecution of the Pagans a long time ago, but that is past and it won't happen again

15) What do you know about the history of Christians persecuting/killing/slandering Wiccans/Witches? Do you think they are justified in some of their actions? What do you think about the way Wiccans are treated by some major Christian institutions (the Catholic Church)? [offer explanation and examples of religious persecution]

It makes me feel bad for the the Wiccans, but they are not a real religion so the church must have some reason. I think instead of persecuting them we should educate them.

16) Describe a stereotypical witch.

She has long black hair, pale face, and has long nails. She is dressed in black, wears lots of jewelry and makeup, and keeps to herself.

17) Have you ever heard of a Catholic Witch? What do you think about them?

No.

[Explanation of a Catholic Witch]

They are confused and wrong. They are not Catholic at all and should be educated.

I-Search: The Modern Witch Hunt

Lauren Brown

As a Wiccan, or Witch, I have had to deal with discrimination and ignorance about my religion. Wicca or Witchcraft is one of the fastest growing religions in the country today. Yet, there are countless acts, many of them legal, of violent, discriminatory, or unconstitutional actions taken against Wiccans each year. Our society is ignorant about Wicca and the discrimination that is going on against us. In this paper I tried to inform people about basic Wiccan beliefs and some of the major acts of discrimination against them. Discrimination against Wiccans is something that I have experienced first hand and an issue which needs to be discussed openly.

Because Wicca is a religion that is often misunderstood and misrepresented I knew that I would have to provide my readers with general background information and history on the religion. I started out by going to various well known Wiccan web sites to get general history. The web site that I got most of my general information about is "The Witches' Voice: A News & Education Network." (*The Witches' Voice*. Feb. 1997. The Witches' Voice Inc. 6 Nov. 2000. <http://www.witchvox.com/wvoxhome.html>.) This site has information on Wicca written for people who know little or nothing about it. If offers some history as well as many links to other sites. Along with this web site I used the book *Witches* (Eisenkraft-Palazzola, Lori. *Witches*. New York: Smithmark Publishers, 1999.) In this book I found general history on Witches in general, including information on Celtic, Greek, and other cultures that had witches in their belief This book also offered a brief glance at the history of persecution of witches. I also used the book *Drawing Down The Moon* (RavenWolf, Silver. *To Ride A Silver Broomstick*. St.Paul: Llewellyn Publications, 1997.) This book gives a very in-depth look at the history of Wicca and gave me the info I needed to complete my brief history on Wicca.

After completing my history on Wiccan and the general beliefs of Wicca I needed to find out the modern history of Wiccan persecution in the United States. To do this I used information from the Alternative Religions Religious Education Network *(http://www.aren.org/.* Visited on Nov. 15). This site provided background information on the constitutional rights of Wiccans as well as some of the court cases that have legitimated Wicca as a religion. I then used a collection of articles that I had gathered from newspapers and online newsgroups to provide examples of specific events that had happened recently where Wiccans were discriminated against. I used the Fort Hood situation as one of my main examples. At Fort Hood, Texas (a military base) a group of Wiccans started a group (with permission of the military) and are being persecuted because of their beliefs by the community and government. Christian groups are spreading rumors about the Wiccans of Fort Hood eating their children and killing animals among other things. Some people in the government are also taking action against the Wiccans, including Presidential candidate George W. Bush. I also used examples about Wiccan teenagers being suspended from school for wearing Pentacles (a five pointed star surrounded by a circle, representing the elements making up life and the higher power), and putting hexes on teachers. I took another look at the schools by writing about how Ms. Shari Eicher, a public school teacher, lost her job because her name appeared on a Wiccan web site. I also wanted to include personal experiences in my paper. This is an important part of the article because it gives it depth. To do this I did not have to do any research other then to back up my facts. I picked out some of the more important causes that I have helped with. I am including the law case that I consulted on (although I can not list specific details as of now, such as names, dates, and locations), problems I had in high school, and a situation I had when applying to college.

After finding out current issues involving Wicca I decided that I should talk to someone who has the opposite perspective of the situation as I do. I think that Wiccans should have the same religious rights as anyone else and we should be protected by the first amendment. I managed to find someone on campus who was a devout Catholic who believed that Wicca is not a religion and that we are just polluting the moral system of America. I interviewed Audrey B. (name has been changed) on 11/18/00. During the interview she stated that: "Witches don't believe in God. They worship the Devil and they don't believe or care about heaven." and, "No [they do not deserve the same legal rights as Christians]. They are not practicing a real religion, so they should not have religious freedom or any of those things. They are not on the same level as us [Christians]." This interview let me know what beliefs and practices of Wicca I would have to discuss in my paper. This interview helped me to narrow down my topic more and let me know what I should focus on.

After the interview I really had the focus for my paper, but I still needed to link it to the UVM and Burlington communities. My first reaction was to write how accepting both of these communities are. Burlington in particular is much more accepting of Wiccans then Columbus, Ohio (my home town) is. The shops in the area and the local Covenant of Unitarian Universalist Pagans (CUUPs) and other covens in the area show how the community lives hand in hand with Pagans and Wiccans. I also wanted to show how the UVM community also accepted Wiccans. Although I decided to stick with the idea that the Burlington community is accepting I changed my mind about the UVM community after a recent Vermont Pagans (a campus organization) meeting. Recently the Vermont Pagans were asked to vacate their office (in the center for Cultural Pluralism) to make room for a faculty member. The Pagans were told this one week before they were supposed to vacate, meaning that the Pagans now have no office, place to meet, or department to be linked to. The reasons were not made clear by the faculty why this is happening. One thing is clear, if a Jewish or Christian based club were kicked out of their building, the University (students and community) would not let it happen. Because we are Pagans, and are definitely a minority on campus, we have to find a new location, something that should not happen. My mind was changed about the acceptance of the UVM community after this incident. I now believe that although the UVM community will not openly discriminate against Pagans and Wiccans, they do not treat them as equals. This then became the main focus of my paper.

By writing this paper I have learned more about the legal rights of Wiccans as well as accumulating more information on the injustices that have been recently committed against Wiccans. It also let me see that although the community may say they accept everyone they don't necessarily follow through when dealing with certain minority groups. My search has turned out well. I gathered information that a person that knows nothing about Wicca will be able to understand and will provide them with ample background information. I think that when people read my paper they will see that there are injustices being committed against a group that has been misrepresented by culture and society. I hope that people will gain a new perspective of what is going on around them as well as learning what a real Witch is.

The Modern Witch Hunt

Lauren Brown

A typical home, in middle America suburbia. A physician father, a former stay at home mother, two siblings, and a family dog. I may sound like a typical teen, but I am not. I have suffered discrimination because I am a minority.

Why? you ask, because I am Wiccan. Yes, that is right, I am a witch. At the age of twelve I started studying the peaceful, pagan religion of Wicca. I am a witch, but I do not believe in the devil, I don't sacrifice animals, I don't eat babies, I don't fly around on a broom, and I do not wear a pointy black hat. Rather, I practice an ancient, nature based religion centered on self improvement and awareness. Although my religion brings me inner satisfaction it often puts me in situations that label me an outcast, cause me to lose friends, or are potentially dangerous. For the past seven years I have faced and fought religious discrimination, a concept that has been outlawed by our government. Although the first amendment claims to protect my religious beliefs, I have been forced to try and find a place where my religion is open and accepted.

When I came out of the broom closet, or became open about my religion, early on in my freshman year of high school, most people still did not know what religion I was. I don't look like your typical "witch." I don't have long black hair, wear black clothing or pentacles (a five pointed star surrounded by a circle), I am do not look goth in the least bit. Rather I blended in with the crowd, I was the stereo typical Ohioain teenager. Usually when people found out about my religion they were, to put it lightly, shocked. Wicca is a religion that few people know about. I would usually receive one of two responses: the "ok, now what does that mean?" response, or the "um, stay away from me" response (a fairly common response).

One time in particular though, I received a completely inappropriate response from a teacher. During Spanish class one day my teacher saw a book in my backpack called *Spell Crafts*. This book had been lent to me by a friend and did not leave my backpack during class. My teacher saw the book in my bag and asked me if I would stay afterwards and talk to her. After class I went up to her desk and her exact words to me were, "Lauren, are you a witch?" I was open with her and told her that I was Wiccan. When I tried to explain what that meant, she responded with, "so do you fly around on a broom in your free time? Do you belong to a coven of *evil* witches? Do you have a black cat, a familiar?" I told her that I did not think our conversation was appropriate and promptly left room. Our school's official policy on the separation of Church and State is that there should be a complete separation. Religion should not be taught or discussed unless it is an appropriate environment. I knew that my Spanish teacher had stepped over the line, but I did not feel safe telling *anyone* about what happened. I did not feel comfortable approaching my parents, friends, teachers, principle, or counselor about the problem because I knew that my religion was not accepted and I feared their reaction. For three years I went partially back in the broom closet, no one but my close friends and family knew or talked about my religion.

During those three years I strengthened my beliefs by practicing with the local pagan community. I gained a Wiccan teacher and became a full Priestess (a practitioner of Wicca) in the eyes of the community. I also started to become involved in campaigns assisting those who had their civil rights violated because they were Wiccan. In the fall of my senior year a crisis broke out at Fort Hood in Texas. The army had placed a large group of Wiccans there so they could practice together. The local community, as well as commanders on the military base, started rumors about the Wiccans on base. Rev. Jack Harvey has mounted a crusade against these Wiccans/Witches. He attempted to prevent the Wiccans from practicing their religion on the Army post. Rev. Harvey said, "These people are demonic, we don't say they might be."

Rep. Bob Barr, R-Ga. agreed with Harvey. Barr tried and failed to outlaw Wiccan practice on military bases. "This move sets a dangerous precedent that could easily result in the practice of all sorts of bizarre practices being supported by the military under the rubric of religion." Barr wrote to Fort Hood's commander, Gen. Leon J. LaPorte. "What's next? Will armored divisions be forced to travel with sacrificial animals for Satanic rituals? Will Rastafarians demand the inclusion of ritualistic marijuana cigarettes in their rations?"

My Wiccan teacher, Heather, asked me if I would write an editorial for our paper, The Columbus Dispatch, to 'let people in Ohio know about the problem.' I wrote a letter to the editor, and it was published. The next few weeks of school were hell for me. Although my government teacher thought that the article was a great step for a high schooler to take, my other teachers reacted with an air of contempt. Three copies of the New Testament were taped on my locker in two weeks. I received pamphlets stuffed in my backpack and my locker about how to save my soul, and how to convert to Christianity. Jokes, looks of hatred, and flat out name calling were whispered behind my back and spoken to my face. I went to my counselor, and he told me that I should have expected a reaction like this. I went to my parents and they told me it was a life lesson, and maybe I should consider becoming a different religion. I went to my friends, and was met with closed ears.

By the last month of my senior year most people had forgotten about the editorial in the paper. That is when things flared up again. A boy in my school, named Paul, decided one day that he was going to preach outside school by the flag pole about his faith, Lutheranism. He printed up t-shirts that said "I believe in Paul" to advertise his sermon. Students as well as teachers started to wear the shirts two weeks before his planned event. Soon he started handing out papers that told people how to "make it to heaven." These papers were also distributed in class by teachers. When these events started I found that many students were unhappy what was going on. They knew that it was a violation of their civil liberties, but they did not want to make a scene and be considered outsiders.

By this point in my high school career, I had decided that I was sick of people discriminating and persecuting people of other religions. I called the ACLU and talked to Heather. They recommended that I contact the local media, talk to my principle, and if need be preach my own sermon about the first amendment and accepting people of other religions. During the next week I appeared on the news three times as an "upset teen witch." I spoke to my principal, with a group of students, about the teachers wearing shirts and pamphlets, and he informed us that he would speak to them. Everything started to look better when teachers stopped wearing the shirts and passing out information, and even though Paul was allowed to preach outside, he was not allowed to advertise in the classroom anymore. Everyone who had been involved in stopping Paul's sermon had decided that we would go to the event and ask educated questions to show other students that we did not approve of his methods of conversion. Soon though, things turned for the worse.

Monday morning, three days before the sermon, I received an anonymous letter in my locker. It said "Jesus is watching you, you will pay for what you have done." I immediately took the note to my counselor and principle, but was told that it was not really a threat and nothing could be done about it. Throughout the next two days I received many comments in the hall that were of a threatening nature. I went home that night and told my mother what had happened. This time she supported my cause because she felt that my first amendment rights were being violated, but she could offer me nothing more then the option of staying home if I did not feel safe at school. I knew I could not flee the situation because people were counting on me to be at the sermon and voice my opinion. I had to stand up for those who were afraid. The day of the sermon I went to school and although I was scared, I knew I had done the right thing. I went to the event and asked my questions, and made my point. Although my last week of high school was unpleasant and uncomfortable, I am glad with the choice I made.

I survived high school and I survived Ohio. I knew though, that when I went to college I would need to find someplace that would accept me for who I was. A place that would accept my beliefs, a place where I could feel safe. One of the reasons I came to the University of Vermont was because the Vermont Pagans, a campus organization, was respected among Wiccan groups in Ohio. Another reason was because of the good reputation of the local Covenant of Unitarian Universalist Pagans (CUUPS). When I came to UVM I had high hopes, that have now been injured. The Burlington community as a whole is very accepting of Pagans and Wiccans, but, the UVM community has proven itself not to be. UVM prides itself on its acceptance and accommodation of minority groups, but this is proven to be false. A few years ago the Vermont Pagans were the "pet project" of the Center of Cultural Pluralism. They took the Pagans in and provided them with an office and meeting space. Recently the Pagans were told that they must vacate their office by December 1st, to make room for faculty. This means the Pagans have nowhere to go, until they can be accepted by another department. Although not all the reasons are clear of why the Pagans are being removed from their office one thing is clear, if the University ever tried to do this with a Jewish or a Christian group, there would be problems (i.e. protests). Because the Pagans are a small and fairly new group and cannot defend themselves and the University is free to kick them out as they please.

Throughout my experiences as a Wiccan in modern society, I have learned many things. I have learned to be proud of my beliefs and stand up for what I believe in. I have learned that if you cloak yourself in secrecy others will suffer. I have also learned that although I am guaranteed first amendment rights by the constitution our society will not allow me to practice my religion safely, openly, or with confidence. I also know that although a place may say that they are open and accommodating it can be a front for the outside world. Underneath they can and will push about those who cannot defend themselves. The most important thing I have learned though is that I can never give up looking for a place where I can be Wiccan and be proud of it.

History of Witch Hunts

1215 Excommunication of Witches

1486 The Malleus Maleficarum, "The Hamme of the Witches," written by the Dominican Kramer and Springer is used in the inquisition

1542 The first statute against witchcraft in England was passed by Parliament

1563 A new statute against witchcraft was issue under Elizabeth 1, ordering the death penalty for witches, enchanters, and sorcerers.

1603 King James of England declares Witchcraft a capital crime.

1688 Salem Witch Trials

1727 Last official burning of Witch in Scotland

1736 Repealed the Witch Act of 1603 with a declaration that Witchcraft does not exist

1915 A Witch is stoned to death by a mob in Texas (last known murder)

1951 Last Witchcraft law repealed in England and replaced with the Fraudulent Mediums Act.

1985 Witchcraft is recognized in the United States.

1999 Persecution and violence escalate against Wiccans at Fort Hood, Texas.

1999 Ms. Shari Eicher, a public school teacher must quit her job because of discrimination and threats that started when her name appeared on Wiccan web site.

2000 Presidential candidate George W. Bush declares: "I do not think witchcraft is a religion and I do not think it is in any way appropriate for the U.S. military to promote it."

2000 Girl in Tulsa suspended for putting a hex on her teacher.

Some Basic Wiccan Beliefs:

*"Wicca is a loosely organized pagan religion centering toward reverence for the creative forces of nature, usually symbolized by a Goddess and a God." (Scott Cunningham, Wicca: A Guide For The Solitary Practitioner)

*All of the major Wiccan celebrations occur on significant events in nature such as, solstice equinoxes, and full moons. These holidays celebrate life, birth, fertility, purification, the harvest, and many other things.

*Wiccans do practice magick (the "k" is to distinguish it from parlor tricks). To Wiccans, magick is just like praying. It is the projection of natural energies to produce needed effects.

*No matter what type of Wicca someone practices, they always believe that religion and life are closely tied to nature.

*Wiccans believe in the Law of Three "For everything that you do, it will come threefold back to you."

*Wiccans do not practice animal sacrifices!

*Wiccans do not believe in Satan.

*Most Wiccans believe in reincarnation.

*The Pentagram or a *five* pointed star (with point up) with a circle around it, is often the symbol used for the Wiccan religion. It is not a Satanic symbol. It can represent the elements needed for life (earth, air, fire water, and spirit) with Spirit being the top point to represent Spirit over body.

Thirteen Goals of a Witch

(According to Scott Cunningham)

I. Know yourself

II. Know your Craft (Wicca)

III. Learn

IV. Apply knowledge with wisdom

V. Achieve balance

VI. Keep your words in good order

VII Keep your thoughts in good order

VIII. Celebrate life

IX. Attune with the cycles of the Earth

X. Breathe and eat correctly

XI. Exercise the body
XII. Meditate
XIII. Honor the Goddess and God

Self Evaluation

Lauren Brown

When we started this assignment I had a general idea of what I wanted it to be on, Wicca, my religion. I knew I wanted to do my paper on Wicca but I did not know how to approach the topic or link it to the community. Doing the research process, and draft revision process helped me to chose a topic and point of view that I think made a strong point and a well written paper.

My final draft definitely has strengths coming from the point of view, and the voice. I wrote it from a personal point of view, one of a person who has been discriminated against because they were a minority. I tried to show throughout my paper how I went from hiding from this discrimination to fighting it. I also talked about how I was searching for a place where I thought I would be accepted, UVM. The voice in this paper is very strong (i.e. "Yes, that's right, I am a witch. At the age of twelve I started studying the peaceful, pagan religion of Wicca.") This was a strength because it gave a more personal look at the topic.

One weakness of the paper is that I wish I could have incorporated some more data and facts in my paper and not just in the side bars, this includes snippets of my interview. I tried to do this but the final project turned out to be way to long so I had to cut it down a bit.

I started this draft about five different times. Each time I would go back over what I had written and decide that it was too "please pity me" or not strong enough. When I started writing my current draft I decided to start off as portraying me as a typical teen: "A typical home in middle America suburbia. A physician father, a former stay at home mother, two siblings, and a family dog." Once I had written this first sentence the paper just started to flow.

After I wrote the paper I went back and added in facts, quotes, and other bits of research. I then wrote the side bars. The two of the sidebars took a lot of research. The "History of Wicca" side bar is just a list of dates and events and the "Basic Wiccan Beliefs" is just a little bit of what I originally had. I had trouble writing "Basic Wiccan Beliefs" because there is just so much to say.

This paper is the hardest paper that I have written for this paper. Although the research was interesting, it was hard to incorporate it in my final draft. It was also hard to take such a personal stance on something that I am still trying to accept in my own life. Overall I think that I did a good job on my last draft. I worked for a long time to find the voice and perspective that I wanted to take on the draft, and I think the final product was successful.

Research Topic Letter

Ryan Corlis Trombly

Dear Professor Turner,

The research topic I have decided to focus on is the issue of Seasonal Affective Disorder (SAD). Seasonal Affective Disorder is the disorder that causes severe depression during times of bad, and dreary weatherto those diagnosed. Many people have and are being diagnosed now after the disorder's discovery. Those who are inflicted are rendered unable to function normally; they have no energy to function, no ambition to even go on, and not even enough concentration to complete a single task. As the name implies the effects of the disorder are seen only in seasons of bad, dreary weather, and is more commonly observed in areas where the seasons dramatically change to or that are constantly in rainy, cold, and snowy weather conditions when sunlight is scarce.

This is an interesting topic to me for several reasons; a couple of them being that I have personal experience with the fairly newly discovered disorder, and also that I have interest in one day becoming an epidemiologist and the research of the incidence, distribution, and control of this disease relates quite well to that field. I was thinking that this topic would relate to the local area very well as this is an area of drastically changing seasons that definitely experiences a season of bad, dreary weather. I thought it would be helpful to speak with Professors from the University of Vermont Psychology Department for scientific information concerning the disorder, as well as to speak with students and residents of UVM and the Burlington area who may feel the effects of this disorder. I am unaware of what causes this disorder physiologically and am very interested to find out, and also I'd also like to see how many people are affected by this and to what extent these people are affected by the disorder.

Annotated Bibliography

Ryan Corlis Trombly

1. Bower, B. "Bright lights dim winter depression." *Science News* Oct. 24 1998: 260.

This article in *Science News* magazine focuses on the medically accepted therapy for treating Seasonal Affective Disorder, light therapy. It tells of the scientific aspects of the disorder and the research that supports and disproves the field of Mental Health's most commonly used treatment of it. It clearly explains the accepted reasons for the depression caused by the deprivation of light to the body in times of darker and drearier weather like in areas that endure long and cold winters or long and cloudy rainy seasons. In writing the self-help guide, that will be my research paper's focus, this is a good source to the legitimacy of science's cure for the disorder and it's effectiveness in treating it.

2. Brauer, Dorothea. Personal Interview. 20 November 2000.

Although I have yet to interview Dorothea Brauer, a counselor at the university's Counseling Center who is very knowledgeable with SAD, I expect to get a lot of useful information from her in regards to Seasonal Affective Disorder in a college setting. Especially information in concern with here at the University of Vermont that witnesses drastic changes in seasons and the climate, and the effects of a dark and dreary winter season. I plan to perform a survey asking students on campus about how the seasons affect their moods and how they cope with times of bad weather. With these I feel that a solid connection can be made for my research paper to the local area, and also to the university and the additional stresses that college can add to the symptoms of those who already face the affects of seasonality. A large portion of my self-help guide to fighting Seasonal Affective Disorder in a college setting should come from these valuable sources.

3. Rosenthal, Norman. *Winter Blues*. New York: Guilford, 1993.

Norman Rosenthal is by far the top authority on the subject of Seasonal Affective Disorder. He first discovered the symptoms of the ailments related to the disorder twenty years ago at the National Institute of Mental Health. He has been presented many awards and honors for his work in the field of Mental Health and with the disorder, and has performed and published the most research concerning the possible causes and remedies to SAD. His book *Winter Blues* is the complete handbook on the topic and covers information from how St. John's Wart can act as a natural anti-depressant to ways and activities that will help cope with the transition of seasons and the depression caused by it. It will be a good asset in writing my research paper for numerous reasons. He discusses the disorder at an everyday level as he details every aspect of the symptoms, reasons, and therapies of SAD. In constructing my research paper my plan is to direct the focus of the paper on a self-help guide to fighting the ailments of seasonality in a college setting where many other stressful aspects may add to spans of depression. This book will be an excellent reference for understandable and accurate information to writing the guide.

4. *Health Oasis: Mayo Clinic*. 12 Nov. 98 *<http://www.mayohealth.org/mayo/9602.sal.htm>*.

This website from the Mayo Health Clinic is by far the most in depth link to information concerning Seasonal Affective Disorder. It covers the history of the disorder, the general information concerning the disorder, and most importantly for writing my self-help guide to fighting seasonality, people and ways to seek help for problems related to the symptoms of SAD. It will be a strong reference piece for factual and statistical information.

Also it is connected to the Mayo Health Clinics main web page, that contains a multitude of many more studies and writings that focus on more detailed aspects of the Seasonal Affective Disorder, many of which are field studies on the topics and more concerned with managing seasonality in everyday life settings.

5.Wegscheider-Hyman, Jane. *The Light Book: how natural light and artificial light affect our health, mood, and behavior*. New York: Ballantine, 1990.

Jane Wegscheider-Hyman's book on the treatment of seasonally and environmentally caused depressions takes a look at the ways light can enhance our moods and better our health on an everyday level. She inspects the medical and personal treatments and methods of treating Seasonal Affective disorder with light and covers common ailments related to the light deprivation. Her discussions of the use of artificial and natural light to treat SAD, and other related disorders, is clearly valuable to my research for writing my guide as it tells of the numerous ways light can negatively or positively affect our lives everyday, and what we can do to control it.

Interview

Ryan Corlis Trombly

Interview Transcript: Dorothea Brauer

Q.) What are the symptoms of Seasonal Affective Disorder?

A.) As light becomes less available symptoms that can occur, as you might have read in my article in the Cynic, they can have sleepiness, fatigue, increase craving for carbohydrates, a lethargic feeling. With this they can lose focus and it's hard to concentrate on tasks, can't do work and can get feelings of depression. They sleep more in the winter.

Q.) Who is likely to suffer from Seasonal Affective Disorder?

A.) There hasn't been a connection made to certain ethnic groups, as sickle cell anemia is a characteristically African-American disease, no connections have been made like that. It is more prominent in colder climates. Women do seem to have higher incidents though, in the same latitude it's like 25% women to something like 17% for men who have SAD. There hasn't been enough research done on that though. The closer to the equator the less incidents occur.

Q.) Are people who suffer from any other form of depression more likely to also suffer from Seasonal Affective Disorder?

A.) SAD isn't related to depression, not seasonally affected, people who have depression are going to suffer more severe symptoms during winter months. Severe sensitivity to light has an effect.

Q.) Is the Burlington area an ideal setting for the onset of Seasonal Affective Disorder?

A.) Yes, Burlington is a very cloudy city. People can feel SAD in the summer too. People can feel hypomanic in the summertime, feel much more awake and will lose sleep. They feel they can do anything and that they have all the energy in the world, become irritable, impulsive. Some people lose their jobs due to bad behavior in the work environment. Your job matters, the more stressful the occupation the worse for SAD. For someone like a salesperson this could be good in the summertime and bad in the winter, keeping up with clients that is. They'll be active and work hard in their jobs during the summer and in the winter when they get lethargic they'll stop returning calls and things like that. Here in Burlington compared to around the equator that is 12 to 12 day and night, we have long days. Some people with SAD need less light in the summer than they're exposed to and more light in the winter. Need to be careful of light exposure. Burlington has high incidence though, in Denver that is cold too it's much more sunny there are less incidence there.

Q.) Would students who come from nicer climates that come to UVM be more likely to suffer from SAD with such a drastic change in environment?

A.) With the people I talk to that are from nicer climates I see that they have a hard time adjusting. They don't understand where there depression is coming from. They aren't used to weather affecting their moods.

Q.) Do the stresses of college life add to the problems associated with SAD?

A.) Stress is a big factor! Need to live as stress free as possible

Q.) How many students (%) would you say suffer from SAD?

A.) Couldn't give you a percentage, but around *25–30%* are affected to some extent by SAD in the Burlington area. Symptoms vary a lot for everyone.

Q.) Could SAD drastically affect a student's life here at UVM?

A.) SAD can definitely affect a student's life at UVM. They won't be able to function well, and it would be hard for them to keep up with the work load. It can really have a negative affect on students.

Q.) How severe can the symptoms related to SAD become?

A.) It could very well lead to Manic Depression, suicide could be a possibility but isn't common. The person would probably already suffer from depression.

Q.) What are some everyday things that a UVM student could do to avoid the symptoms of SAD?

A.) Plenty of exercise is important, need to stay active. Need to avoid carbohydrate binging, need to go outside even if it's cloudy. More illumination outside than inside. If this doesn't work they can use the light we have at the Counseling Center, if they start using it a lot and see that it is beneficial than they need to buy their own. We usually have them come in and use it for a period of time before classes or something to see if it helps.

Q.) Where could someone go to that feels they might be suffering from SAD here at UVM? Who could someone that feels they have SAD talk to for help? What are some treatments that can help a UVM student.

A.) The Counseling Center here at the University of Vermont has counselors who can discuss SAD and light therapy with students. We have a free light that students can try to see if it helps. Medication and light therapy are used to treat serious cases. Have them come in and use the light for a period of time each day to see if it's effective. Can also take it to see if it helps with studying.

Q.) Are there any prescription medications or other forms of treatment that can help those inflicted with SAD?

A.) Severe cases are treated with anti-depressants if light therapy doesn't work.

Q.) Is there anybody on the campus of UVM doing research on the subject of SAD currently?

A.) No one's doing research on SAD that I know of. The Counseling Center is planning to do a survey this winter some time, maybe in January, just asking people certain Likert scale questions. Like 1 to 10 if you feel that you agree more with a statement, the more you agree with it the higher number you circle, you know? Asking questions about light, how often, how much, things of that nature. Asking questions about how light affected them this winter.

Dark Day, Better Days: Seasonal Affective Disorder (SAD) and the University of Vermont

Ryan Corlis Trombly

"Spring passes and one remembers one's innocence
Summer passes and one remembers one's exuberance
Autumn passes and one remembers one's reverence
Winter passes and one remembers one's perseverance"
—Yoko Ono, *Season of Glass*

Matthew Ruttenberg's only ambitions were to successfully settle into his freshmen year at the University of Vermont in the fall, after receiving his letter of acceptance to the university in the spring of his senior year in high school. He nearly tore the mailbox apart everyday, after recklessly speeding into his driveway, in hopes of finding the letter that would answer a multitude of questions that had riddled his head for the past few months. It had been a long, stressful and emotional senior year, with the seemingly endless hassles of academics, social activities, and tentative college plans that he faced everyday. He now could take a breath of relief; he relaxed in the past four years of high school memories and rejoiced over the numerous opportunities that now awaited him at college in the fall.

The summer days of Hialeah, Florida went fast, anticipation and ambition being a large part of the reason for this. Before he knew it, he was sitting alone in his stark 11' by 13' dorm room that was now home, his mother's farewell embrace still engulfing him. He was now at the University of Vermont with infinite goals and the fresh ambition to achieve them. He loved the fresh mountainous air and the clean, vibrant green lawns that stretched across the campus, a far contrast from his urbanized, lowland hometown that sits just outside of Miami. As the sun set over Lake Champlain and the Adirondacks he couldn't help but think about what tomorrow would bring.

As his first semester began, he was energetic, focused, and most of all ecstatic to be at the University of Vermont. Although it was a difficult adjustment to make he did it with ease; he was surrounded by conciliatory fellow students who he found easy to befriend, the work load in school was at first overwhelming but he expected it and was doing well, and he enjoyed the constant activity of the college life. He had settled in and was forming everyday patterns to manage his valuable time. He was extremely content with his life at the University of Vermont; after all it had been his top choice since visiting the school the summer before his senior year in high school. The one and only thing he disliked as the year carried on was the sharp breeze that blew more and more foliated leaves from the trees each day, and that stung his face more and more each morning as he walked to class. He knew Burlington's characteristically bitter winter was fast approaching, but he still thought little of it except that he would definitely have to get used to the cold weather.

He had never endured more than a day of frigid weather, let alone months of it, but as the temperature slowly dropped with the passing of each day he knew that he would now have to. All had been going well for him and he saw no barriers in his way, but he was starting to feel the wear and tear of the hectic college lifestyle and schedule. Late into the semester he began to drag; he just didn't feel like his old self. He began to feel sluggish it was even difficult for him to finish daily calculus assignments that he had little problem with earlier in the semester. When friends stopped by to see what he was up to or to ask him to do something he'd either be sleeping or he'd irritably tell them "nah."

He started to oversleep classes, even if they were at 1p.m. in the afternoon, and the back load of work quickly piled up. He would sleep for more than half the day, and when he was awake he'd wish his lifestyle would allow him to sleep more. Eventually he secluded himself in his room only leaving to grab foods that he was craving at Simpson Hall (Brauer). The farther the sun slipped behind the dark foreboding clouds that cast a shadow over Burlington, the more he isolated himself in his dorm; he never suffered from any depression before, and just blamed it on the being homesick and being overloaded with school work.

As with 25–30% of people living in the Burlington area, my roommate, Matthew Ruttenberg was suffering from Seasonal Affective Disorder (SAD). He had never before dealt with the climate having an effect on his mood, and had a hard time understanding why his decline came about (Brauer). For centuries, sunlight has peaked and dwindled throughout the year, creating seasons that biologically affect humans in numerous ways. Seasonal Affective Disorder (SAD) is a product of this, causing a mood disorder that is associated with the seasonal variations in light (Mayo Clinic). As Burlington skies became more and more overcast, and the natural light of the sun depleted my roommate became increasingly symptomatic to the affects of SAD on his everyday life, and setting back the clocks on daylight savings time hadn't helped. I have seen the affects of Seasonal Affective Disorder (SAD) with both family and friends, growing up in the not-so nicer winters of southern New Hampshire, and even brought the subject up to him. He just exclaimed that it wasn't the case, and to be honest, I didn't know enough about it to convince him that it might be.

I decided to do research, hoping I'd find something in text that would force him to look into the subject more for himself. For years I've listened at the dinner table as my parents discussed how my uncle couldn't hold a job because every winter he went through a "funk" and even heard them talking about how he was getting treated for SAD. I can also recall a few of my friends saying they suffered from it, but still I didn't know much more about it than maybe a few characteristic symptoms. I hit the books and found a lot of information, some dry and way too scientific for me, and some that was both interesting and useful.

It was clear to me, after researching for a while, that there would be plenty of information that might grab my roommates attention and that might prove helpful to him. I found that even though scientists and greater thinkers, like Hippocrates and Socrates, have contemplated the relationship between the mood and season since as far back as two-thousand years ago, substantive research on the matter went neglected until a renewal of interest in seasonal forms of depression was brought about by Norman Rosenthal, MD and colleagues at the National Institute of Mental Health(NIMH) in the early 1980s. Rosenthal, considered today the top authority on SAD, along with colleagues at NIMLJ had been conducting research on seasonal depression through the study of seasonally affected patients, who seemed to me to be much like Ruttenberg, and discovered that melatonin secretion (the excess being the cause for SAD, as I later told my roommate) could be suppressed by bright artificial light with positive results for the patients tested.

This breakthrough motivated Rosenthal to carry on with more extensive research and in 1984 he authored the now classical research paper in which he identifies and describes Seasonal Affective Disorder (SAD) for the first time. Rosenthal was able to validate SAD through clinical and demographic features, and responses to a specific treatment that he had considerably helped to discover, phototherapy (Malan and Canguilhem 77-78). From Rosenthal's extensive and innovative research and findings on the disorder, numerous scientists decided to also research the matter and its form of treatment, worldwide.

I found that as with Matthew Ruttenberg, thousands upon thousands of people suffer from the mood disorder, SAD, every year with symptoms as minor as irritability and lethargy to as severe as manic depression and suicide. Seasonal Affective Disorder (SAD) has been epidemiologically proven to be largely affected by region of habitat, as Ruttenberg found out, with studies showing that 1 in 10 people in Alaska and 1 in 100 people in Florida that are affected by this disorder (Bower 260). Burlington, and the University of Vermont for that matter, is an extremely cold area to live in the winter much like Alaska. More importantly, Burlington is also a cloudy and dark area to live during the winter months similar to Alaska (in lesser terms), with short days and little natural light. For this reason Burlington is an ideal region for the incident of this disorder, and due to the facts that Ruttenberg is unfamiliar with the climate's affect on his mood and that he is already burdened by the stresses of college life, he is an ideal candidate to suffer from it (Brauer).

I gathered the produce of my research and hurried back to our dorm room in hopes of catching my patient before he left for his daily trip to Simpson Hall to eat. Right as he was walking out the door I berated him with information. He merely asked me if I wanted to join him, which seemed to me like the perfect opportunity to grab his attention. As we sat down for Crossroad Burgers and pasta, an odd but often seen combo with our friends for dinner, he actually opened up to what I had to say, perhaps moved by my concern. To my surprise it was the physiological reasons behind the problems Ruttenberg and other sufferers of SAD faced, that he really found interesting. With each bite he read more and more about how Rosenthal and others discovered that SAD were due mainly to the ill effects of the hormone melatonin and its relationship to light. I merely sat by, occasionally pointing out things like how melatonin is a hormone produced by the pineal gland, which is involved in sleep regulation and biological rhythms, and that the hormone when secreted into the bloodstream has been proven to cause body temperature to drop, a factor characteristic of sleep. The relation between light and melatonin (as discussed earlier) is that "the amount of light seems to determine how much pineal melatonin is actually released from the pineal [gland] and secreted into the bloodstream." He read out loud with a long voice, "The more light, the more melatonin release is suppressed. The less light, the more melatonin the bloodstream carries. Light suppresses melatonin release" (Lindsley).

What this all means for people like Matthew Ruttenberg is that during the winter months that are notably severe in the Burlington area, fewer hours of light occur. This means that the period of time that melatonin is being released into the bloodstream is increased, and therefore, logically, the actual amount of melatonin in the bloodstream is increased. Falling asleep is associated with lowered body temperature and waking up is associated with an increase in body temperature. For many, including Ruttenberg, this drop in temperature caused by excess melatonin secretion that is associated with falling asleep is the cause of their loss of pep, loss of energy, sluggishness, and eventually depression. A majority of people are not affected by the melatonin levels in their bloodstreams, but those like Ruttenberg that suffer from the symptoms of SAD are (Rosenthal and Wehr 672).

It seemed now that he was convinced, as he quickly asked me how they treated it. We found together an article that discussed how the original therapy for suppressing the symptoms of SAD, and still the most commonly used (even though controversial to some scientists), is Norman Rosenthal's treatment of phototherapy, now called bright light therapy (BLT). He found great interest, as a lover of the Classics, in the fact that treating depression with light dates back as far as two-thousand years ago when Greco-Roman physicians treated it with light from the sun and oil lamps (Malan 79). Today after numerous studies, many supporting and some negating its effectiveness, BLT is still thought to provide the best remedy for SAD. The BLT consists of exposing those suffering from SAD to bright artificial light (2500 lux) for two to six hours a day. This is supposed to suppress the melatonin from being released and therefore the symptoms caused by too high levels of melatonin in the bloodstream (Wegscheider-Hyman 113), It's effectiveness for curing symptoms is usually seen after three to five days and in sixty to eighty percent of patients treated with it (Malan 79).

Although it has been proven to be effective many scientists still question whether BLT is an aid physiologically or mentally. Still to this day biological mechanisms through which bright lights produce anti-depressant relief remain poorly understood. Some scientists just believe that if it works, use it. Psychologist Anna Wirz-Justice of the Psychiatric University Clinic in Basel, Switzerland states that "light therapy should be considered a mainstream anti-depressant [therapy]" and "that light is as effective as [anti-depressant] drugs, perhaps more so" (qtd in Bower 260). The University of Vermont Counseling Center, who aid people like Matthew Ruttenberg with SAD problems during Burlington's long winter, has a bright artificial light that they use as treatment for SAD. They too are studying its effectiveness with those that use it, but have so far reported positive responses supporting the use of BLT as a treatment for SAD (Brauer). Other treatments for SAD are anti-depressant drugs, and with severe cases the combination of this with BLT. Orally administered melatonin has also been contemplated for regulating SAD patients sleep patterns, but still faces much skepticism. It has also been researched for the usage as a sleeping pill, with much publicity and little success (Lindsley).

As we walked back to the dorms, through the torturous cold, Ruttenberg asked me what I thought he should do, and who he should call here at the University to see if treatment might be helpful. The next day I decided to call the Counseling Center where I spoke to Dorothea Brauer, a counselor and significantly knowledgeable person on the subject of SAD. She answered my questions thoroughly, as she told me how Burlington is an ideal setting for the onset of SAD during winter months. She went on to state that numerous students at UVM, don't recognizing it (like Matthew Ruttenberg) or that think that there's nobody here that could fix their problems. As my roommate and I found, and that Dorothea Brauer confirmed, is-that SAD can really prove to be a serious detriment to those students' academic performance and social lives, and can even ruin their college experiences at UVM all together. It was emphasized that there are people that can help though, and that the Counseling Center of the University of Vermont have plenty of great counselors who can discuss students problems with SAD. They are equipped with artificial bright lights and are more than willing to let UVM students try bright light therapy (BLT) for a period of time before classes or to borrow it to study, in hopes of bettering study habits and overall living quality. If BLT is ineffective than they would then discuss possible medications of anti-depressants with those suffering from SAD. I was glad to relay this information to my roommate as he arrived from classes, and was even more satisfied by his immediate phone call to speak with Dorothea Brauer.

If any student at the University of Vermont has questions concerning Seasonal Affective Disorder (SAD) then they can contact the Counseling Center, located at the corner of Main Street and South Williams Street, by phone at *656-3340* between the hours of 8a.m. and 7p.m. Monday through Thursday or 8a.m. to 4:30p.m. Friday (Brauer). Seasonal Affective Disorder (SAD) can be overcome, and perseverance can be had, you just may need some help in doing so.

It was quite clear to all who knew and saw my roommate, Matthew Ruttenberg, on an everyday basis, that he was steadily adapting to the bitter winters of northern New England that hamper so many peoples' moods. He was the same person I met during summer orientation after returning from winter recess, and his sunny home in Florida. The second semester, even more dark and cloudy than the first, proved to be an enjoyable one for Matthew Ruttenberg. His academic performance and social life came alive, and the University of Vermont, which he loved so much and then despised even more, finally became a comfortable home and good choice in his eyes. The Counseling Center and the bright light therapy proved effective in remedying his problems with Seasonal Affective Disorder (SAD), which so many other students also face. I have to admit though, that I think a big part of his turn around came from the sheer fact that he knew what the problem was, and how to address it, thanks to me!

No one should have to suffer the problems associated with SAD here at UVM, like Matthew Ruttenberg did. There are various ways for students like him to prevent the symptoms related to SAD here at the University of Vermont:

- Students need to pay close attention to their energy levels and mood.

• Stay physically active; go play basketball at Patrick Gymnasium, ride a bike along Burlington's bike path, walk to and around Church Street, anything that gets you out and active.

• Stay away from carbohydrate (starchy, sugary foods) binging. That means less spaghetti at Harris-Millis and less beer drinking, even if you crave it.

• Get outside even if it's cloudy. There's more illumination outside than inside. If there is a need to stay inside let in plenty of light from the windows and light the room as well as possible.

• Manage time well, and keep a strong mind. Overcome the daily stresses of the college lifestyle.

• If symptoms related to SAD persist and they begin to negatively affect your happiness and daily activities seek professional help. Don't be ashamed or try to hide it, there are plenty of people at UVM that want to help you. (Brauer/Wegscheider-Hyman 124-125)

Seasonal Affective Disorder (SAD): Works Cited

Bower, B. "Bright Lights Dim Winter Depression." *Science News*. Oct. 24,1998:260.

Brauer, Dorothea. Personal Interview. 20 November 2000.

Health Oasis: Mayo Clinic. 12 Nov. 98 *<http://www.mayohealth.org/mayo/9602.sal.html>*.

Lindsley, Gila. *Seasonal Affective Disorder (SAD): About light. Depression & Melatonin*. 18 Nov. 2000. *<http://world.std.com/-halberst/contrlb/sad.html>*.

Malan, Andre, and Bernard Canguilhem, eds. *Living in the Cold: International Symposium*. Montrouge: John Libby Eurotext, 1989.

Rosenthal, Norman F., and Thomas A. Wehr. "Seasonal Affective Disorder." *Psychiatric Annals*. 17.10 (1987): 670-674.

Wegscheider-Hyman, Jane. *The Light Book: How Natural Light and Artificial Light Affect Our Health, Mood, and Behavior*. New York: Ballantine, 1990.

Bibliography

David

Prescribed Burning: Should We Do It?

http://r05s001.pswfs.gov/stanislaus/five/burning.htm. Accessed 11/12/2000

This page was part of the USDA Forest Service website. It describes briefly what is involve in prescribed burning, what the ecological importance of it is, and why the Forest Service does it.

http://www.tncfire.org/manual/sitemap.htm. The Nature Conservancy's Fire Management Manual. Accessed 11/12/2000.

This manual has good explanations of the requirements that this organization holds for conducting prescribed burns.

Franklin, S. (1999). Prescribed Fire Litigation. *Wildfire,* v 8, p 19(3).

This is a short article which is fairly pro-prescribed burn. It discusses the importance of prescribed burning to trees and understory organisms. It also outlines some of the cost/benefits of prescribed burning. It seems like it should have some good, basic information that will be helpful, such as how much prescribed burning costs per acre.

Kost, M., DeSteven, D. (2000). Plant Community Responses to Prescribed Burning in Wisconsin Sedge Meadows. *Natural Areas Journal,* v 20. p 36(10).

Although this article is about sedge meadows in Wisconsin, I thought that it would be important because Vermont bogs are rich in sedge plants. This research article follows the results of experiments dealing with burning and the use of ash to treat overgrown sedge areas.

Smith, J. J. (1986). "When Let-Burn-Fires Get Ready to Roll, Campers Hit the Trail." *Smithsonian,* v17, p 42(11).

This is a journal article about exactly how fire is able to regenerate forests. It uses lighting fire management in Montana as its main example. This should be of use because it talks about tree succession regeneration as it pertains to fires, set or natural.

Tiedmann, A., Klemmedson, J., Bull, E. (2000). Solution of Forest Health Problems with Prescribed Fire: Are Forest Productivity and Wildlife at Risk? *Forest Ecology Management*, v 127, p 1(18).

This journal article gives a description of what the effects of burning, prescribed and non-prescribed, has on forest ecosystems as a whole, not just on tree populations. The article uses the Blue Mountains of eastern Oregon as an example. Although it does not pertain directly to Vermont, the rules for coniferous forests apply to all coniferous forests.

Fighting Fire with Fire: Interview

David

I interviewed Dale Bergdahl of the University of Vermont's School of Natural Resources:

What degrees do you hold, and from what institutes?

Doctor Bergdahl got his bachelor degree in forest management at the University of Minnesota. He received his Masters degree and PhD from the University of Minnesota's Plant Pathology department.

What is your experience with prescribed burning and forest fires in general?

He has spent two summers in Idaho as an undergraduate working on fire related projects and has used prescribed burning to treat dwarf mistletoe disease among conifers, black spruce in particular.

How do you use prescribed burning to treat diseases?

Dr. Bergdahl said that the way they treat such a disease with burning is by clear-cutting an infected stand, then burning off all underbrush to destroy all infected saplings.

Is prescribed burning practiced in Vermont?

Dr. Bergdahl attested that prescribed burning is used in Vermont but not nearly as much as in other areas of the country. It is used mainly to control populations of unwanted hardwoods and for the control and management of berry crops.

Is the impact of burning on an ecosystem different from system to system, and if so, what is the importance for Vermont forests?

He said that yes, the end result will always be different because you get different results depending on what you begin with. Its importance for Vermont forests is mainly in fuel consumption, he said that "people did not introduce fire to the ecosystem". It is a natural phenomenon.

Is prescribed burning used in Vermont for sedge growths?

Dr. Bergdahl said that prescribed burning was mainly used on the forests of Vermont, and to an extent as an alternative to herbicides as a herbaceous-plant controller.

Exactly how does prescribed burning help revitalize soil?

For the most part prescribed burning returns nutrients held up in standing trees to the soil. Ash and phosphorous are the more important things that are returned to the soil.

How does fire, natural or set, aid in plant succession? I am under the impression that it acts as a sort of "reset" for forests, returning them to the first stage of plant succession?

He said that yes, after a long time (several hundred years), starter organisms in the succession cycle would become rare, and that fire can act as a sort of reset, allowing the first plants to establish a population again by opening up the area.

Does prescribed burning have a goal, that is, should it eventually become unnecessary once it has returned the forest ecosystem to a cycle of natural burning, or do you believe that it will always be used by man to keep forests in balance?

He said that prescribed burning will always be used as a means for fire management.

How effective is prescribed burning at stopping out-of-control wild fires?

I learned that the process of using set fires to burn off fuel to prevent the movement of wild fires is called "backfiring", not "prescribed burning"

Has the above-mentioned practice contributed to the recent jump in the number and size of wildfires?

Dr. Bergdahl said that absolutely the suppression of wildfires by the U.S. Forest Service for the last 10 decades has contributed to the buildup of dead organic fuel and the explosion of wild fires this year.

Do you think that many people understand that fires are necessary for the proper functioning of ecosystems?

Bergdahl seemed very convinced that the vast majority of people do not understand that fire is absolutely vital to ecosystems. He referred to forests as "adapted fire systems". He believes that the "Smokey the Bear" mentality is still very alive with the public

How can it be changed?

There need to be more regulations regarding building in the back-country. Bergdahl said that there are more and more people building homes in remote areas, and they have to understand that those areas WILL burn, especially in the west. He said that the U.S. Forest Service has guidelines for backcountry structures to make them more fire-resistant

Do you have any other thoughts about this subject in general?

Dr. Bergdahl asserted that education of the public is key, he said that they need to be willing to pay (taxes) for fire control and management NOW or they run the risk of paying in the future with lost land, lives, forests, and rising insurance costs due to property damage from wild fires. He concluded that we have to "manage fuels today so we don't pay the cost tomorrow".

Fighting Fire with Fire

David

The rain falls steadily, creating a soothing, rustling sound as it strikes the tree canopy. Two inches fall in one night, completely drenching the forest. The crew awakens from their sleeping bags the next day, the morning sun slowly sucking the high peaks out of the dark. The deep green forests glow brilliantly in the early morning light. Looking over the miles they have covered in previous days, several members of the fire crew spot another plume of ash gray smoke, right where they were just 24 hours ago. The thin column transforms into a massive cloud, completely engulfing one mountain in a mere half hour. It is soon apparent that the crew is right in the fire's intended path. The crew leader blares commands over the CB-radio. The crew awkwardly scrambles to the safe zone, a several-hundred yard area of clearing. Sitting in the center, they watch a week of work, hours of sleepless labor, burn up in a few hours. A Sikorsky helicopter screams overhead, trailing behind it is what looks like an oversized child's pail attached by a heavy-load cable. The massive bucket contains over 700 gallons of water. The crew is thankful that they have made it to the safe zone; if there is one thing more dangerous than the fire, it's the water. 750 gallons of water directed at a pinpoint location will kill a person just as quickly as the fire will.

This was not at all an uncommon scene in the western United States in the year 2000 fire season. During this particular season, close to eight million acres of forest burned in the United States, in contrast to the usual annual norm of two to three million. This drastic increase forced president Clinton to approve the use of U.S. military to aid in the war against the fires. The situation got so desperate that forest-fire fighters from many other countries had to be called in as backup, according to Chris Casey, a fire worker who spoke recently at the University of Vermont's School of Natural Resources. The year 2000 fire season was the most intense that the U. S. Forest Service has ever seen. The reasons for such problems and the solutions to them are intricately linked to fire itself.

Forests are, as Dale Bergdahl of the University of Vermont's School of Natural Resources said, "adapted fire systems". If you study the way a forest forms and the trees and shrubs that compose it, you will notice a pattern. This pattern is more specifically called plant succession. What happens is that for one reason or another, an area of forest is cleared by: heavy wind or ice storm, a volcanic explosion as with Mt. St. Helens, or, as is most often the case, a forest fire. Once an area of forest has been cleared, reforestation begins almost immediately, even though the signs of it cannot be seen for years. The first trees to populate a recently cleared area are fast populating trees that thrive in open environments. Pines and aspens are both very good at this, and both have their own mechanisms to deal with surviving fire. Pines not only repopulate devastated areas very quickly, often forcing their way in due simply to their overwhelming number of seeds they produce, but they are also one of the only trees with a fireproof reproduction system. There are many pinecones produced by each tree, each containing multiple seeds. Of all these pine cones there are a few produced that are not only fireproof, but also activated by heat. These few pine cones will only open and release their seeds when exposed to heat. They will lay dormant until a fire comes through, and after the fire has passed, they pop open and release their seeds. Aspens survive fire in another way: when the upper section of an Aspen burns, the roots stay alive. Shortly after the fire has passed, the roots from just one tree will immediately send forth hundreds of aspen seedlings, right out of the old root system.

Saplings of such trees, however, have trouble surviving for many generations. As the forest grows, the new seedlings and saplings are forced to grow up in an increasingly shaded environment. These trees are thus called "understory intolerant". At this point, more understory tolerant species will move in, and eventually, as the original generation of pines dies off, will replace them as the dominant species. This can be seen in many forests all over the country, even in Vermont. One can walk through a conifer (cone producing trees, like pines) forest and see that the seedlings are mostly oaks or maples. These seedlings can survive and even thrive under the shade of larger trees. This is how the forest grows, evolves, and how every species gets its chance to exist there. Fire is necessary to reset the cycle in some areas. When a fire sweeps through an area, it gives those fast-establishing species a chance to repopulate the area once again. Fire is absolutely vital for the survival and health of forests.

Fire plays another very important role in the survival of forests. As a forest ages, the original plants that established it will die off. Then the next generation will die, and the next. They are constantly replaced with new seedlings, however the dead material will build up. That dead material becomes dry and very combustible, at which point it is called fuel, and unless something regulates their concentration, they can fuel massive infernos that will engulf hundreds of thousands of acres in a very short timeframe. Nature's solution to this problem was to deprive forest fires of the fuel necessary for them to get out of control. Forests burned for millions of years before human kind came along, as Dale Bergdahl put it "people did not introduce fire into ecosystems". Up until the U.S. Forest Service started forest fire suppression around the turn of the century, nature had used frequent, small fires to burn off built up fuel. However, for the past hundred years, the U.S. Forest Service has been suppressing forest fires, so for the past hundred years, fuel has been building up to dangerous levels in the United State's forests. It had become a literal time bomb. The Forest Service could extinguish and suppress fires as long as they stayed with reason. Of course, more fuel built up as a result of the fire suppression, and the fires kept getting bigger and bigger, because they had more fuel to work with. It was only a matter of time before the fires got too out of control to stop. This year, three times the acreage burned than has burned in most average years. This was not the case here in Vermont, both because Vermont tends to be moister and has not experienced as much fire suppression as the west has. Fire suppression is not the way to deal with this problem, as the problem arose from suppression. Rather the answer is prevention and containment.

Forest fires are prevented these days by prescribed burning used along with other methods. Prescribed burning is essentially the use of human started fires, strategically placed, to burn off dead fuel. The goal is to eliminate the fuel, but not to allow the living trees to catch on fire. Thus prescribed burn sites are meticulously monitored to make sure that a "runaway fire" does not occur (Franklin). Prescribed burning is very effective as a means of preventing large scale blazes by eliminating fuel, however, it has many other practical uses.

Nutrient revitalization is one of the big benefits to prescribed burning. Burning has served for millions of years to return some nutrients to the soil in forests. The suppression of forest fires by the U.S. Forest Service over the past ten decades has contributed to the poor health of forest ecosystems in the U.S. When organic material dies in a forest, it takes a very long time for it to decay, in fact, it can take over 100 years for a large log to completely decompose. This slow decomposition slowly returns nutrients to the soil, which is what support seedling growth between fires. However, periodic fires are necessary for quick boosts of nutrients, which help give seedlings an advantage in gaining a foothold (http://r05s001.pswfs.gov). Fires not only free up nutrients in fallen trees, but also in the "litter" or fallen organic material, such as pine needles. "fire exclusion from forests is often said to result in steady accumulation of litter and stagnation of decomposition and nutrient recycling process" (Tiedemann 7). Tiedemann continues to say that "frequent or repeated burning has been suggested to release nutrients" (7). Essentially, without fire, nutrients would not return to the soil fast enough, however, too much fire can be a bad thing. A healthy combination of slow and fast nutrient revitalization is best for forest health.

In Vermont, prescribed burning is used as a means of fuel consumption, fire prevention, and nutrient revitalization; however, it has many other uses, many of which are directly related to timber industry and agriculture. Prescribed burning is often used by the tree harvesters and farmers of Vermont, particularly berry farmers. Timber harvesters, to eliminate unwanted hardwoods from their stocks, use prescribed burning. For example, a pine harvester does not want oaks or maples, which are more competitive in the understory than the pines seedlings, infiltrating their crops. To eliminate this problem, timber harvesters will apply low intensity burns to the understory. This will burn only the seedlings, but not reach high enough to ignite the adult trees. Harvesters can then supplant pine saplings in areas that have been cleared.

Aside from being used for agricultural purposes, prescribed burning can be used to eliminate the presence of certain diseases in pure stands (a stand is simply a forested area, a pure stand being an area that consists solely of one species) of trees. In my interview with him, Dale Bergdahl recalled his usage of prescribed burning to control dwarf mistletoe disease amongst black spruce. He said that when an infected area of a stand is located, the entire section is cut down, then the understory is burned, because the seedlings and saplings, being the offspring of infected trees, will also be infected. This form of control works very well for containing and eliminating a disease, especially in valuable timber crops.

Farmers also use prescribed burning for the control of unwanted plants. Prescribed burning is a very beneficial and environmentally conscious alternative to herbicides. Farmers who want to clear out unwanted weeds and other invaders from their crops may use burning because it is cheaper than herbicides, and it is less controversial, because unlike chemicals it leaves no residues on food crops. It is also less environmentally detrimental, and it directly returns nutrients held up in the weeds to their crops. It is, in many situations, a superior alternative to chemicals.

It is absolutely vital that the general public have a better understanding of how important fire is and why the forest service must let fires burn sometimes, in what are called free fire zones (Smith). The Forest Service is moving towards, and has been since the 1970's, a system of fire containment, but not fire suppression. However many people do not understand the significance of this. As Dale Bergdahl feared, more and more people are moving into the backcountry, and few of them know the risk involved. He stated that while the Forest Service produces a list of guidelines for fireproofing backcountry homes, people have to understand that their home will not and cannot always be saved if fire gets out of control. Bergdahl is very convinced that people have to be prepared to accept the cost of managing the lands. He said "the public needs to be willing to accept the cost of managing fuels now or we will all pay the price tomorrow (in lost land, life, forests, and insurance costs)". This is very much true, it only costs between \$15–\$1500/acre to prescribe burn as a means of fuel management. On the other hand, to suppress an already out of control wild fire, it costs up to \$1 million per 24-hour period of fire suppression (Franklin). Plus, large western forest fires can easily cause billions in damage to homes and to the forest itself. In the long run, fuel consumption is less expensive, better for ecosystems, and less expensive for the taxpayer.

Education is the key to this whole issue. One of Dale Bergdahl's biggest concerns was that the "Smokey the Bear" mentality is still alive in the minds of the American public. This old belief that fire suppression is the way to go is simply wrong. Hopefully, education by the U.S. Forest Service and by individual members of the scientific community will aid in informing the public of what the situation is and what needs to be done about it. People need to realize that fire is not a bad thing, and that it is absolutely necessary for the survival, balance, and health of forest ecosystems. The public needs to learn to live with fire, because suppressing it will only compound the problems for future generations.

Alive From Beneath

How a Small Store's Character Brought It From Tomb to Tops

Michael R. Dorta

The saffron railing leads below into the cold, dull concrete cave. The descent is steep and narrow as the steps sadly slope to the left with age. It is the submersion into a perilous coal mine. Never knowing what the chilling darkness holds below. The railing assures you to stay on course. The concrete that closes in around you forces your hands to your sides, never wanting to touch the cold dirty death that plagues the walls. A dim glow looms around the corner and breaths from within. Something's alive and begging you to make the deep plunge within. Something draws you in; asks you to go beneath the surface.

Scott Bellows was lured into the Pure Pop record store three months ago by this same means. He now works there and enjoys every minute of it. Being forty-one years of age, Scott isn't the typical teenager working at a chain music store in the mall, trying to make money the easiest way he knows how. Scott is in it for the music, the people, and the atmosphere. All of these combine to offer what he feels is the "hub of working here," he promises me. Around these fine aspects, Scott centers himself within the store and enjoys one of the most "interesting cross-sections of environments," he says with eyes beaming and thoughts running deeper. This "cross-section" is what Pure Pop is most popular for; whether this pertains to its musical selection, its customers, its employees, its 1600 square feet of store, or the overall atmosphere. But Scott reassures me that the best asset to this store is the staff. "We have young and old employees, over flowing with musical ideas that they are dying to share. We have classical people, Jazzy, Trance, anything and everything—just not that mainstream crap," he assures me smiling and searching me with his eyes, making sure I didn't take offense to that.

Whereas most music stores look for what's the most popular or "mainstream" at that time, Pure Pop refuses to. According to owner John Crandall in an interview with the National Association of Recording Merchandisers (NAIRM), "Instead of concentrating on hit product, we try to look for and anticipate developing markets."

When I asked Scott what kind of character he thought this "underground" setting gives to the store, he actually drew a direct correlation to not only the employees, but the customers as well. Brow narrowed and thinking hard, Scott explains himself, "Being new to Vermont, I've noticed that Vermont marches to it's own drummer—this store does the same thing." It's this linkage that provides the integral aspect to this store. Pure Pop is not like the "cookie-cutter" chain stores that we are so accustomed to today. This independent store is as original as it gets. The old ceiling tiles sag lower and lower, while the poles throughout the shop exert all their force back up in response. It is their last line of defense, and the struggle for existence is fierce and continual. The wooden shelves and files scattered everywhere hold the CDs. Wood that may once have given birth to splinters now is infertile. With so many hands running over them in the past, the wood has been reduced to a cardboard-smooth surface; giving each shelf character and differing shades. The concrete walls of this bomb shelter are bathed in purple in an attempt to disguise the hideousness. The water and ventilation piping run like yellow veins against the purple backdrop in an effort to make them stand out so much, that they actually become invisible. The contours and cartography of the basement floor are all visible despite wearing a thin rug for a mask. The whole room appears to be a makeshift environment, yet this is what gives it the character that is unmatched in any other store. Just like the customers and employees, so different but everything comes together to create an atmosphere where anyone feels comfortable and can fit in. The chains that restrict and conform a store's freedom of thought do not fetter pure Pop. As the owner, John Crandall explained in an interview with NARM that, "We try to be the grass roots of what's new in music for our customers. We're not built on selling hit product."

Listening intently, but trying not to appear to be doing so, Casey Forbes, another Pure Pop employee, is eager to be part of anything that is going on in this store. Almost before I can ask him. Casey so friendly answers yes to doing an interview. Avoiding eye contact, you can tell he might be a bit insecure. But when something that he knows a lot about comes up, like music or the store, you can be sure he will excitedly answer your question immediately and directly at you. At 24, Casey is one of the youngest employees and loves being part of "the Niche" he calls Pure Pop. He says customers feel this atmosphere too, especially the "college students from places with strip malls. This is Burlington's version of a record store, and they grow to like it. We get a lot of regulars."

He also said that he has been on the other side of the business. Casey used to work at Borders. But there were so many people working there and it was so impersonal that he believed no one would even recognize if there were "regulars" to the store or not. Even though large chain businesses like Borders and Sony can be proud to report operating revenues of 56,621,825 dollars in 1999 (1 Sony), Pure Pop has a deeper mentality and Philosophy: please the customer, please the employees and listen to music. Casey describes how, "We don't reach out and try to draw the people in, Pure Pop draws them in effortlessly." Although it may be difficult to think of how such a small business can make a name for itself against a multi-million dollar corporation, Pure Pop is no longer a secret. In 1995, Pure Pop won the Single Store Independent Retailer of the Year Award according to the National Association of Recording Merchandisers. Quite an achievement when you realize how the business started out. In 1980, John Crandall opened this tiny shop in the basement it remains in, and it consisted of approximately 3,000 albums, which was originally his own collection. In an interview by NARM Crandall admits, "It was really painful at first to trade and sell them, but I consistently used the money to reinvest in new product, and we slowly grew from there." "Slowly" is hardly the word to be used, when a store about the size of six dormitory rooms gets noticed nationally as the best independent music store in the Nation. This is simply unheard of. But with the unlikely yet unique and exciting setup and a crew that makes the whole store glow with warmth, it is somehow a bit more tangible to us.

Casey eagerly describes how coming to the store is like an adventure; you come down the steps, and fully enjoy hunting and foraging for music stuff. He says this in a manner where I'm surprised he didn't run up the steps and reenact this.

Many may say this is as a story of David and Goliath. Yet I believe that Pure Pop is not aiming at the giants. Instead it is going about its own way not even paying attention to the punches that the giants are attempting to land on them. As a result the store keep rising and rising while the Goliaths try to keep up. And this is what makes Pure Pop the victor and the chains the defeated.

Pure Pop may be a bit hidden in a tomb-like basement, but it is alive from beneath. It can truly be felt by the generous and down-to-earth attitudes of both the employees and of the underground shop itself.

Works Cited

Bellows, Scott. Personal interview. 7 Nov. 2000.

Forbes, Cohn. Personal interview. 7 Nov. 2000.

"Pure Pop: Single Store Independent Retailer of the Year." *NARM: Sounding Board (1995):* 1-3.

Sony Music. 20 April 2000. 1 Nov. 2000 <http:\\www.world.sony.com/R/Financial/ARI1999/Highlights.html>.

Stick it in Me and Make Me Beautiful

Debi Budnick, Alayne Donka, Pete Murphy

ACT 1

Deb: So did Tim call you?

Alayne: No, not yet. I'm still waiting.

D: You could wait for the rest of your life. You should move on.

A: But I heard he was going to ask me to the prom.

D: This Cosmo magazine says that the best way to get a guy to ask you to the prom is to play hard to get.

A: That's what I've been doing. It doesn't seem to be working. Speaking of prom, are there any good dresses in that magazine?

D: I dunno man. These girly magazines are pretty wack. They never really have anything useful, except that I need to lose 20 pounds.

A: The boys are so cute though.

D: Yea, most of them. Except for this one!

A: Ahh! That's kinda weird.

D: Why would somebody do that to their body. It says here that some cultures in West Africa pierce their upper lips and then stick these plugs in there. The bigger the plug, the higher the status. (Ebin '79)

A: Why would they have something like this in Cosmo?

D: I dunno. It's just an article on body piercing.

A: It's not usually what comes to mind when I think of body piercing.

D: Yea, really. It's one thing to pierce your nose, but this is a little much.

A: It says here that he uses the horns of a beetle to make him look fierce. (Ebin '79) Well I don't want anything like this, but I am thinking of getting a piercing.

D: Alayne, what's wrong with you? What happens if it gets infected?

A: It won't get infected. I'll take care of it.

D: Well where are you thinking about getting this hole in your body?

A: I dunno, maybe like a belly button ring or in my eyebrow. What do you think?

D: I think you can do whatever you want. And I also think that Tim is not going to take someone to the prom with a big, bloody, peeling, nasty scab on their body.

A: Well if I get my belly button pierced, he may not be able to see it.

D: Well I should hope he would. It is prom night.

A: Deb, I'm not a big slut like you.

D: At least I'm not the one that's gonna end up looking like this guy.

A: I'm not gonna go that extreme.

D: Well I should hope not, in this society these piercings are used to distinguish adults from their seniors. Your tits do that already.

A: I just want to get a belly button ring. Why can't you support me in this.

D: I don't support you because you don't have a good reason for doing it. At least these people have good reasons for getting these piercings. Like check this out: the Suya of Brazil got their ears pierced because they thought it helped them hear better and understand more. What's a belly button ring going to do? Cure your flatulence? (Brain '79)

A: Well if that's what it does, maybe you should get it. I just want it because it will look cool with a bikini.

D: Why not something less permanent like booby tassles. Do you even know anything about belly button rings?

A: I know that like every other girl has them, and I want one. Why is this so hard to understand.

D: Well, you can do what you want. But just make sure you have a good reason.

A: Well its not like I'm gonna go to the first scummy place that I see to get it done.

D: No, you're gonna go to the second or third or the fourth. All those places are scummy.

A: Have you ever really been to a piercing studio?

D: Hunny, people create art in studios. They don't put holes in each other.

A: Body piercing is a form of Art.

D: Says who?

A: I read about it in Time. This one anthropologist did an entire exhibit in the Museum of Natural History in New York. Body art is one of the oldest forms of art. People use body art as a form of expressing themselves just like photography or painting or ceramics. But, they use the body as their canvas. (Lemonick '99)

D: You read Time?

A: You know I have really been seriously thinking about this. I am glad **you** think this is funny, but this is something I want to do. I think I am going downtown to talk to somebody about this.

D: Well, I am sure you can convince me that it's cool. But what about your parents?

A: I'll work on them later, after I get all my facts straightened.

D: Let me know how it works out. In the meantime, how do you think this dress would look on me?

A: Well if you're going for cheap and trashy, you're all set. Otherwise I would keep looking.

D: Glad I have friends who can be honest with me.

ACT 2

Pete: Hey, can I help you?

Alayne: I am thinking of getting my belly button pierced. But, I kinda wanted to find some information about it before I get it done. Do you think I could ask you a few questions?

P: Sure, whatever you need. I really suggest that you set up an interview with your piercer before you get it done.

A: Alight, thanks. How long have you been doing piercings?

P: Hmm, a ways back. Probably for about 7 or 8 years.

A: Is the naval piercing thought to be a pretty painful piercing, or is it usually pretty harmless?

P: It really depends on the person. I have had people in here that have had a really bad time of it, but a lot of people think the whole process is pretty easy. (Teresa Lorenco, Nov. 19, 2000) Let me ask you a question though. What is your reason for wanting to get pierced?

A: I just think it looks cool. Its really as simple as that. Why do a lot of the people that come in here get a piercing?

P: Many get it for the same reason as you. Some get it done to give them individuality. It can be the same thing as when you put on a certain clothing in the morning. For me, it separates me from everyone else. It also is sometimes a right of passage, like for something victorious. But, overall, I guess it is just a simple passion for me. (Jason Pratt, Nov. 16 2000)

A: I can agree with all that, but I feel pretty sure that I want to get this done. The only thing I am concerned about now is how safe it is to get pierced.

P: Oh, not to worry, I will give you whatever information you need. I am confident that we use the best technology and the safest means when we pierce someone.

A: Well what steps exactly do you take to make sure that I am safe?

P: Here, we use a medical autoclave to sterilize every single piece of equipment and stuff that is used when I pierce. What this does is expose our tools to extremely high temperatures to a point where all bacteria are killed. We also use single-use needles, so no infections or disease can be spread that way. All the jewelry is sterilized and is either surgical steel, gold or niobium.

A: Well that sounds reassuring. One question that I have always had though, is why would I want to come here and have my piercing done with a needle instead of a gun.

P: The two methods are really completely different. What the needle does is extract an area for a ring to fit into. It leaves nothing behind so the wound can heal naturally. The gun, on the other hand, is just a puncture. It forces a stud through the flesh, usually leaving a flay of skin behind causing the wound to get infected. One big difference that you should be interested in is that the gun is not sterilized. Places can't put the gun into the autoclave because it is plastic and would melt, so you are not kept completely safe from disease.(Jason Pratt, Nov. 16 2000)

A: Well that is really good to know. I am glad I didn't go to another place first.

P: Yea, not to worry. To tell you the truth, it honestly won't affect me if you get you piercing done here. I like to look out for my customer's best interests. So I will be straight up with you. You can check all around town if you want, but I guarantee you that you are safest to get your piercing done with the methods we use. As long as you take care of your piercing afterwards, the whole experience will be completely harmless and safe. But whatever you choose to do, remember these safety measures.

A: One last thing though. What about the healing process?

P: Okay, well, generally it take 6 months to 2 years to heal completely. You must make sure that you don't touch your piercing and that you wash it once a day with anti-bacterial soap. You must never use alcohol swabs, Betadine or hydrogen peroxide to clean your piercing. Stay away from spas and take care of it when you are in a pool. To help the healing process, you can take vitamin C and zinc. The jewelry should not be changed until the piercing is healed. (Dr. Richard Janus, 1999-2000)

A: Oh, definitely. I would get it pierced right now, but I need to think about it first. I will hopefully be back though.

P: Okay. I hope to see you soon then. I am glad you took the time to find out about the piercing.

A: Thanks for your time. It was really helpful. Wish me luck. Bye.

ACT 3

Antionette (Toni): Steve, get in here! Get off your fat, beer drinking, lazy ass and get in here.

Steve: What the hell could you possibly want during the fourth quarter of the division championships?

T: Look what our daughter is going to do to herself! I found this in her room when I was putting her socks away.

S: She puts her own socks away.

T: Well then I was vacuuming.

S: We have a cleaning lady.

T: Okay okay. I was snooping. Regardless. It doesn't matter. Look what I found. I think she is going to get her naval pierced.

S: Well what the hell is she doing that for? I'll be dammed if I am gonna let that happen while she is living under my roof. Alayne, get down here!

T: Steve, we have to stop her. I can't take it anymore. I am a failure as a mother.

S: Take it easy Toni.

A: What do you want?

T: My baby, why, why? I gave you everything a mother could!

A: What are you talking about? What did I do? Am I grounded?

S: Don't play those games with me young lady! Your mother found *this* in your room!

A: What were you doing in my room?

T: Cleaning, and don't talk back to your father.

A: You haven't cleaned in years! That's Rosalita's job.

S: That's beside the point. Lets get serious here. The piercing is out of the question.

A: It's my body, it should be my decision!

T: I carried your body in my stomach for nine months, not to mention the 3 days it took you to get out! I think I have some say in this too!

A: Its not like I'm just going to jump into this. I've actually done some research. This is a big decision, and I've been thinking about it for a while.

T: What makes you think we are going to let you do this?

A: I am almost an adult, old enough to make my own decisions, this shouldn't be a concern for you guys.

S: Key word there is almost. State law says you have to be 18, or you need our permission, and I'll be damned if I'm gonna give that to you. (Lorenco, 2000)

A: You haven't even heard my arguments yet!

T: Fine, go ahead then, lets hear what's so important.

A: First of all, it looks cool.

S: Who the hell is going to be seeing it young lady????

A: People will be seeing it in the summer when I wear a bathing suit, old man!

S: Not if I don't let you out of the house they won't.

T: Steve, cmon. You think it looks cool? What kind of a reason is that!

A: Why else would people get it done?

T: Well, you read that magazine. That tribe in Brazil use it as a right of passage. I thought your Bat Mitzvah was enough! Also, it said that the jewelry worn can show status. (Brain, 79) Do you want people to know your father is a urologist!

A: Well did you see the part about the Native Americans? They used piercings as a form of identification, to express themselves. (Grinde 2000). I think that's a better reason than anything. If you are going to do something like that to your body, it should be for personal reasons.

S: It may seem cool to your generation, but most people your mothers age still see it as social deviance, because it is still a sub-culture. You're obviously doing this as an act of rebellion (Pratt, 2000).

A: What? What are you talking about? Since when do urologists know what a subculture is? Get your head out of your patient's asses for a second and realize this is a normal thing now. I'm not rebelling against anything, I'm expressing myself.

T: Well what if it leaves a scar on my beautiful daughters skin! Oy Gevalt. I'm getting all vechlempt.

S: Scarring should be the least of your worries. What about all the blood born diseases like tuberculosis, hepatitis B and E, and HIV? (Jet, 1999). I've seen a lot of nasty stuff in my career, and it's not worth the risk

A: If I go to place that has clean practices, I don't have to be concerned with that.

T: What's your definition of "clean practices?"

A: At Body Art downtown, all the piercers use rubber gloves, and they change them constantly. The never reuse needles, and all the needles are pre-packaged and they open them right in front of you. They use a medical autoclave to clean the jewelry before they use it, and then after they do it, they give you a whole bunch of information on how to avoid infection and make sure it heals correctly. They even give you a number to call in case you have any questions or problems. Is there anything else you'd like to know?

S: Well, maybe that's all true, but what about the belly button specifically?

A: It didn't hurt.

T: What do you mean it didn't hurt!

A: I mean, it doesn't hurt, or its not supposed to anyways.

S: Is there something your not telling us?

A: No, there is something I'm not showing you. But I guess I might as well. I got it done see, Aunt Jenny took me and I did it right and its not infected. HA! Know what else? Aunt Jenny told me about you guys when you were younger.

T: What are you talking about! Steve, get your sister on the phone.

A: She didn't do anything wrong, she only told me the truth. Dad, you had your ear pierced for a month and then took it out. And mom, you told me that nasty whole in your ear lobe is cause you had a mole there! But you actually had an expander!

S: Well I guess there is nothing we can do about it now, she already got it done.

T: I guess you're right, we have to let her live a little like we did. I guess its not that harmful.

S: Just keep those needles away from where the sun don't shine. I don't want the people across the hall in the OB/GYN department telling me my daughter has some nasty infection I don't want to know about.

A: Oh, don't worry, I take good care of that one too.

Bibliography

Abler, T.S. and Einhorn, A. (1998). *Images of native american body modification in the art of benjamin west.* American Indian Art Magazine, autumn, *42-53.*

Brain, R. (1979). *The decorated body*. New York, NY: Harper and Row Publishers Inc.

Ebin, V. (1979). *The body decorated*. London: Blacker Calmann Cooper Ltd.

Grinde. Don. Personal interview. 30 November. 2000.

Janus, Dr. Richard. *Body piercing explained*. 1999-2000. Sydney Medical Body-Piercing Clinic. 16 November 2000. http://www.body-piercing.com.au

Lemonkick, M.D. (1999, November 29). Body Art. Time, Vol.19.

Lifestyles. "If body piercing is so hazardous, why is it popular?" *Jet.* Apr. 1999: *56-69.*

Lorenco, Teresa. Personal interview. 9 November. 2000.

Miller, J-C. (1997). *The body art book: a complete illustrated guide to tattoos. piercings.. and other body modifications*. Berkley Books: New York.

Pratt, Jason. Personal Interview. 16 November. 2000.

Rowanchilde, R. (March 23, 2000). Piercing history and anthropology. [online serial]. (November 2, 2000).http://www.sexpositive.com/SPIweb/essays/production_essays/history_of_piercing.htm

Wilkinson, B. (1998). *Coping with the dangers of tattooing. Body piercing. and branding*. New York, NY: Rosen Publishing Group.

Wojcik, D. (1995). *Punk and neo-tribal body art*. Mississippi: University of Mississippi.

An Illustrative Friday

Draft 4

James Lewis, Andrew Brown

An illustrative Friday in the life of a non-recycler:

•8:00 AM—Wake up and take an extra long shower. Damage Done 25 gallons H20

•8:25 AM—Brushes teeth, leaves water running the whole time. Damage Done = 1.25 Gallons H20

•8:35 AM—Goes to fridge opens half-gallon of milk and pours a cup into plastic disposable cup a la frat-party style. Finishes the cup off and throws it into the wastebasket.

•9:00 AM—Grabs Cereal Bar and heads out the dorm to class in a hurry. Leaves lights and television on in his haste. Throws wrapper on the ground without locating proper receptacle.

•9:55 to 11:45 AM—First class ends and heads back to room to finish a paper. Prints out rough draft of a ten-page English research paper. Makes corrections on computer and prints out final draft. Discards rough draft into garbage bin at the end of the hall.

•12:15 PM—Finishes lunch at cafeteria and chucks whole tray-full of leftovers into the "containers" bin. Buys coffee in a Styrofoam cup and goes back to dorm room to take a nap. Damage Done = Doesn't recycle coffee cup.

•3:00 PM—Wakes up and chews a stick of gum to get rid of bad "nap-breath". Goes to class to hand in paper and spits flavorless gum on the ground. Damage Done = one wad of non-biodegradable occupy aesthetic campus green, or get stuck to the bottom of an innocent bystander's shoe.

•4:00 PM—Rushes back to dorm for executive meeting of the Friday afternoon Drinking Club. Damage Done = six-pack of empty crushed cans never to be recycled and an upset liver.

•6:00 PM—Orders two large pizzas and polishes them off in a matter of minutes. Throws boxes in the paper bin to be recycled. Damage Done = Two UNCLEAN pizza boxes which can't be recycled. Garbage man works longer to filter through rubbish that is not recyclable. Costs UVM $65.50 an hour to sort the garbage.

•9:00 PM—Leaves dorm to go to a raging party. Drinks 12 Genny Lights and throws them in the barrel. Damage Done 450 empties destined for the landfill.

•1:00 PM—Stumbles home dropping a can on the way. Relieves himself on President's bushes and weaves his way to the dorm. Passes out with the lights and television on. Damage Done = 1 can and a slew of electricity.

•1:15 AM—Student sleeps an inebriated sleep oblivious to the disastrous impact he has left in his wake in the mere course of a day.

A typical Friday in the life of an upstanding recycler:

•8:00 AM—Awakens in the morning, smiles and gets out of bed. Being mindful of others takes a quick but refreshing shower to conserve water. Compensates for excessiveness of others.

•8:30 AM—Eats a banana and throws the peel in the compost bucket. It is his turn to empty the compost bucket so he disposes of it its contents behind the cafeteria. A farm that uses it as fertilizer on its crops picks the compost up every other day. Helps out the environment and a local farm all in one fell swoop.

•8:45 AM—Brushes teeth only using water when needed. Water saved 1 gallon.

•8:55 AM—Leaves dorm and goes to shop for coffee. Uses CUPPS (Cannot Use Paper Plastic Styrofoam) coffee mug as per usual. Over 200 Styrofoam cups saved every year.

•9:05 AM—Opens recycled notebook in class and proceeds to take notes. Using one ton of recycled paper saves: 17 trees, 41 kilowatts hours of energy, 7000 gallons of water, 60 pounds of air pollution effluents, three cubic yards of landfill space.

•9:55-11:15 AM—Revises the same English research paper on computer saving ten pages of loose paper.

•12:00 PM—Stays in to make his own healthy, all natural lunch, a sandwich with ingredients already purchased in bulk. Uses own eating plates, glasses and utensils.

Saved: one Styrofoam plate, cup and bowl, plastic utensils, and ? pound of food waste.

•1:00 PM—Goes back to dorm room and collects empty cans and bottles that are redeemable. Catches a ride to grocery store with other students in order to cut back on useless travel and redeems the beverage containers. Uses the money to refill his reusable beverage growlers at the local brewery. Saved: one and a half cases of cans and bottles to be recycled. Implementing the reusable growlers saves another two cases.

•3:00 PM—Makes way to English and stops to pick up a cereal bar wrapper left behind by another less than responsible student. He deftly misses a wad of gum along the pathway . . . close one. Saved: one non-biodegradable wrapper that contaminates the earth and the landscape.

•4:00 PM—After class the student walks back to his dorm and takes a nap after a long night of homework. He is very sure to turn off his computer, lights and stereo. Saved: Costly electric energy that can now be used for a more important cause.

•6:00 PM—Wakes and prepares to walk downtown for a meal in natural foods and vegan restaurant. Saved: Gas, being a precious fossil fuel, chemicals used for fertilizers and pesticides, at least one animal that will live to see another day.

•8:00 PM—After going back to hang out with friends, this student finally utilizes the beverage growlers.

•12:00 AM—Gets ready for bed, picks up the room and places all waste into the appropriate recycling bins. He carefully sorts the garbage from the paper, containers and the salvageable food waste. Saved: a week's worth of accumulated rubbish that may have been taken for granted. Rubbish that may have been disregarded and plainly thrown away.

•12:30 AM—Student sleeps with a clean conscience knowing that he has taken every step possible to reduce, reuse, recycle and save.

At first, these two scenarios may seem to be exaggerated for dramatic effect. However, if one inspected the two lives, one could find them prevalent in most settings and environments. The life of the nonrecycler may not be his fault. There could be a myriad of factors that have added to his atrocious habits. Whether or not his household pre-college recycled is a large factor. The friends that he hangs out with may also contribute to the way in which he acts. In many cases ignorance is one of the largest factors regarding environmental awareness. The demand of time, energy and natural resources often does not enter the minds of people before they make the many choices that face them in a single day. Likewise, whether the second student was brought up with a greater appreciation of the natural world was a factor in his choices. Perhaps this student was active in pro-environmental clubs and groups in his high school. The influence of University level courses cannot be discounted either. If the total net sum of the energy, time and natural resources saved by our model student was calculated for a single day the results should be convincing enough to prove to even the most cynical antagonist that every little bit counts.

Three Generations of Women

Jaime Robertson

"When someone you love dies, you don't lose her all at once; you lose her in pieces over a long time — the way the mail stops coming, and her scent fades from the pillows and even from the clothes in her closet and drawers. Gradually you accumulate the parts of her that are gone. Just when the day comes — when there's a particular missing part that overwhelms you with the feeling that she's gone, forever — there comes another day, and another specifically missing part"—John Irving, *A Prayer For Owen Meany*

This quote stands out in my mind when I think about the deaths of my mother and grandmother. Everyday I learn something new about them, and continue to realize they are gone. But, in a way they are never gone from me. I feel there presence in my life in many ways.

When this research paper was assigned I had some trouble choosing a topic. First, I thought of John Irving, my favorite author, then Van Gogh, my favorite artist. Finally the topic of death just sort of slapped me in the face. Ever since I decided to go visit my Grandmother for the last time, it's been the only thing I really think about. Exploring the topic I have chosen has been very helpful in the healing process. So, when you read my final draft keep in mind that to me this is not just a research paper that I wrote to pass a class. It is a piece of my life that I have finally had the opportunity to explore.

I've been watching my Grandmother die for years now. Not literally, but spiritually. She was crushed by my mother's death in 1982, and she hasn't been the same since, so I've been told. Neither have I. Children finally figure out that some things are constant at about 14 months. This is called object permanence, and the first object known to be permanent by an infant is their mother. Mine died when I was 14 months old and this has drastically affected my life. Her death also touched another life very deeply, her mother's. My mother's life and death has pulled together three generations of women in a struggle that has finally found peace.

Kathie Koplin Robertson is my biological mother. She reached adulthood in a period known as the turbulent sixties.

She was greatly moved by the Civil Rights Movement, Martin Luther King, the Feminist Movement, the arts, and the Beatles. The things she observed in the sixties helped to shape her into the vivacious, positive, and courageous woman she needed to be in order to face the trials yet to come.

The events that took place as Kathie grew up strengthened her desire to help other people cope with trials in their lives. She recognized the hurt in the world through racism and the Vietnam War. In preparation for this goal, she attended Vanderbilt University where she received her degree in psychology. Her involvement in the feminist movement gave her the desire for independence, and she found education to be an answer. She also attended the University of Maryland and George Peabody College in Nashville, working toward her masters degree. During the summers she worked at a camp for asthmatic children, in order to teach arts and crafts to children with whom she had much in common; she suffered from asthma when she was a child (A. Robertson).

The next stage of Kathie's life held many changes. Upon completion of her education, she moved to Springfield, Illinois and worked as a mental health technician at the McFarland Mental Health Center. At this point she met my father, Al Robertson. They dated for about three years and were married in 1979 (A. Robertson).

After their marriage, Al and Kathie began to feel their lives were coming together. Kathie had decided to pursue a degree in nursing, which she completed in 1980. Al had a secure job at a local television station. They were building a house, and preparing to start a family (A. Robertson).

By graduation, Kathie had targeted infant care as her main focus. After graduation, she was recruited and hired by Baptist Medical Center to work in the nursery as a registered nurse. At the time, she was six months pregnant with me. She loved her job and had developed fast friends at Baptist. In February, 1981, she look what was to be a temporary leave of absence to give birth on April 7, 1981 (A. Robertson). The day after I was born my mother wrote in her diary, "Al and I are more in love than ever. He called a million people and is the proud papa personified. I feel so lucky—so happy—so complete."

A month later, my mother was diagnosed with malignant and serious breast cancer. I spoke to my father regarding their reaction to the news and he stated, "We weren't ready for it—

it was a happy time. She had just finished school, we had a new baby. We never ever suspected anything was wrong. However, we were going to beat it. We were going to beat it together." The mass in her breast was found late in her pregnancy, but thought to be swollen mammary glands. When preparing her for treatment, her doctor Jack Stemburg said, "I only know one way to fight this, as hard as we can!"

With the help of Dr. Stemburg, Dr. Bucolo, her nurses, her family, and her friends she began to fight the terrible disease, assuming that she would win. She still had a Woodstock poster. She believed in rebellion, in beating the system.

Despite the difficulty ahead, her hopes were high. When the cancer was diagnosed, it was too large to operate; her right breast was twice the size of her left breast. The doctors began chemotherapy at maximum doses on a weekly basis. The chemotherapy caused extreme nausea. After heavy chemotherapy she underwent radiation. Finally, in October her doctors did a radical mastectomy of the breast. After the surgery there was a renewed hope that there would be healing. My parents' upbeat optimism came from the attitude that their generation could rise to fight any battle . . . and win it. Kathie accepted the inevitable and focused on living every day to the fullest.

Anne Hall was one of my mom's nurses and she describes Kathie during her illness in the following statement, "I think people thought they would help her when they came to visit, but she had so much inner strength, people always left with the feeling they were the ones that had been helped. She gave of herself completely to others. She was always just herself, just Kathie, but being 'just Kathie' was quite extraordinary. If was simply part of her being to always be concerned about others." In speaking to people who were around my mother during her illness I heard statements such as this many many times. She was definitely an unselfish person who gave and gave of herself even in a time of great need.

After she was diagnosed with a terminal disease, Kathie focused on living possibly the greatest fourteen months of her life. "She had just graduated from nursing school and had a brand new baby, but she never once complained" (Al Robertson). She suffered an epileptic seizure on December 25, 1981, my first Christmas. The cancer had spread to her brain.

The hope for recovery was diminishing everyday. In the next few months she stayed home as much as possible. She realized that her time was limited, but focused on life and continued to touch those around her. By spring the cancer had shown up in her bones. In April she went to Slone-Kettering Cancer Center in New York. She was having difficulty breathing, and the doctors found out that it was due to the solidified cancer around her lungs. The cancer had grown back on the chest wall. She was put on oxygen.

Things continued to get worse, and my mother continued to smile. This was a miracle. My dad administered all of her medicine up until May, then it became impossible for him to continue doing so. She required medicine around the clock; he was exhausted. A full time nurse was hired. The pain was so terrible that she was taking 12 milligrams of a synthetic heroin every four hours. On June 24th she asked Dr. Stemburg what else could be done, and he said, "Nothing." She died on June 27th 1982. When I spoke to Dr. Stemburg regarding my mother's attitude toward the end of her life, he said, "At the end she was given a supernatural grace and she shut everything out. She had a tremendous peace. Her lack of fear was amazing."

A hospice program at Baptist Hospital was started in her honor to help others with terminal diseases cope with their lives. Many others grew out of this program. Her memory lives on in those she loved. Before her surgery on October 5, 1981 she wrote my dad a letter that read, "I am so glad to be living and to have so many wonderful people to love. Hugs to everyone. I thank God for you, Al. You are a real blessing. Kiss our Jaime for me everyday. Take her to the beach . . ."

As I have said before, "The loss of my mother at such an early age has impacted every aspect of my life. I learned early that nothing lasts forever; anything and everything could end in a matter of seconds. I knew this before I knew my ABC's, before I could ride a bike. Later in life, this death has helped me to focus on the greater aspects of living. As a direct result of this tragedy I've conquered, I am a woman with character and more love to give the world than I could ever expect in return. I know how to 'plant my own garden, and decorate my own soul.' I am determined to live a full life, to extract all I can out of every situation, and to spread the love I have inside around. The scars I have developed have only increased my strength and heightened my sensitivity" (my last English paper).

Recently, this strength that I claim so often has been tested. My grandmother passed away last Monday. I was down to see her only days before so I got to talk with her for a few days when she was awake and coherent. Up until a few months ago, I knew my Grandma to be a bitter old woman only cheered by her Granddaughters presence. She was very withdrawn from the rest of the family but somehow clung to me as her only link to my mother. We were very close when I was little although she lived far away. After my Grandpa died and she was no longer able to travel as much we saw each other rarely, sometimes only once a year.

This past August, I received a call from Gulf Coast Memorial Hospital explaining that my Grandma was very sick and I should come down. So, I went. I stayed with her in the hospital for about a week. I painted her fingernails, put lotion on her hands, we ate blueberry pancakes (the only thing she ate all week), had a slumber party, and watched *The Horse Whisperer (she really loved* Montana). When I left the hospital for the airport, I thought that it was the last time I would see my Grandma. Unlike my mother, she was not a fighter—she had given up. I can see how life would be less precious with no one there to love you and nothing to do. So, I came to school, sent letters, and called every now and again.

On Monday, November 8th of this year. I received another urgent phone call, but it seemed different this time. She was in a Hospice Program much like the one started when my mom passed away. She wasn't expected to live through the next week. Once again, I went. There was no time for slumber parties or pancakes during this trip. It consisted mostly of watching her sleep, holding her hand, and waiting for her to wake up long enough to exchange a few thoughts and fall back to sleep. She was awake for a while a few times and we talked about my Grandpa, my mom, and her dying. She was beginning to have "hallucinations"—she talked to people who weren't there, but she seemed to be comforted. One moment in particular stands out in my mind. I leaned over to give her a hug and she looked straight up at the ceiling (obviously at something) and said, "I knew she'd come." She was talking about my mother. When I left for the airport this time it was clear that we wouldn't see each other again. I gave her a hug and let her know it was okay if she didn't want to try anymore. She told me to "take it easy" and I left. It was really hard to leave her there alone. I'll always remember her hands; they never changed, and her eyes.

My mother gave me strength to handle this situation, and reflecting on her courage throughout tragedy has inspired me to live in the now. In this time of transition in my life it has been helpful to learn about my mother. It has been an eye-opening experience. Although this paper has focused on death, it has made me believe in living. I believe in planning for the future and I believe in learning from the past. Mostly though, I believe in living. I believe in grabbing each precious moment, making the bad aspects of life faint away, and walking in the present.

I have spent too much time worrying about tomorrow's test, next years elections, and college. I've spent too many sun-lit minutes wondering what non-existent black shoes I'll wear after labor day, dwelling on past exchanges of words that really make no difference, and knowing that I can do better than that. All of my life I've been living somewhere else. I've been dreaming of a future where I'm making a difference, and I've been idolizing a perfect past that never really was. I'm almost never in "today." It was only recently that I realized—Life is what you make it. I do not want to look back on my life from my death bed and regret 8 weeks of living because I was afraid of the very next day. I don't want to see missed chances because the past was my blindness. I want to make little decisions in my life because of how I feel that very second, and decide my evening plans based on what I want to do. I want to stick broccoli in my ear and pretend it isn't there. I want to run barefoot in the rain. I want to plant wildflowers in the snow. Mel Brooks was able to sum it up with his usual witty wisdom when he said:

> Let's have a merry journey, and shout about how light is good and dark is not. What we should do is not future ourselves so much. We should now ourselves more. "Now thyself" is more important than "know thyself." Reason is what tells us to ignore the present and live in the future. So all we do is make plans. We think that somewhere there are going to be green pastures. It's crazy. Heaven is nothing but grand, monumental instance of future. Listen, now is good. *Now* is wonderful.

He's right. Now *is* wonderful.

WORKS CONSULTED

Holleb, Arthur. The American Cancer Book. New York: Doubleday and Company Inc, 1986.

James, Susie. "Group Aids Victims of Long-term Illnesses." *Arkansas Democrat.* 1982.

Koplin, Paulie. Personal Interview. 14–16 November 1999.

Norton, Mary Beth. *A People and A Nation. A History of the United States.* Boston: Houghton Mifflin Company, 1994.

Robertson, Al. Personal Interview. 10 November, 1999 and 14 November, 1999.

Robertson, Kathie. Letter to Jaime Robertson. 8 May 1982.

Robertson, Kathie. Letter to Family. 4 October 1981.

Robertson, Kathie. Personal Diary. 11 September 1980–8 April 1981.

Robertson, Lydia. Personal Interview. 16 November 1999.

Stemburg, Jack. Personal Interview. 12 November 1999.

Stemburg, Maralyn. Personal Interview. 12 November 1999.

Sylvester, Edward. *Target Cancer*. New York: Charles Scribner and Sons, 1986.

Nightmare

Final Draft

Jessica

Last night I had that dream again. I'm a little girl and somehow these two men abduct me. They are carrying me, and laughing. I scream and cry, but no one around me tries to help. I bite into one of these disgusting looking men. The strange thing is that every time I have this dream, his flesh is a mushy consistency, and has the same awful bitter taste. Suddenly I wake up again, and I turn on my nightstand light to jot my dream down in my diary to the best of my recollection. This time I woke up in a cold sweat, but last time I screamed in my sleep, waking my parents across the hall. I'm 14 years old and sleeping at the foot of my parents bed on the floor. They think it's because I like the air conditioning. Really its because I stare into the darkness of my room and my body literally tenses. "I don't want to go in there," I whisper to myself. I take my pillow, my

2

blanket, and for the 37th consecutive night in a row, I curl up in the quilt at the bottom of their bed. My heart is racing as I try to sleep. A song is stuck in my head from some 80's band and torments me. It is by Blondie, "one way or another I'm gonna get you, gonna getcha, getcha, getcha..." Sleep comes.

Oh god I wake up. Where am I? It is so dark. There is a window above me painted gray with the sky. I hear the creak of bedsprings and heavy breathing. I

3

immediately grow sick once I realize what is happening. I wake up to hear my parent's having sex. Oh God, I'm going to throw up. I throw my pillow over my head, and cry.

3 Next night I sleep in my own room, I hear the windows crack, and strange cries outside. My eyes focus on the windows, switching their gaze from one to the next quickly. I think I hear footsteps outside my window crunching on the rocks of our driveway. Oh God, my heart races. I crawl along the carpeted floor of my bedroom and peak out the window. It sounds like someone is playing with my bicycle outside. Oh God it's him, I know it's him. I sink to the bottom of my floor repeating over and over, "God, let it not be, God, let it not be." It becomes more rhythmic then a heart beat, I stare at the walls watching the shadows dance around and deface them. Sleep...

4 I wake up early in the morning, wanting to go jogging but opt not to; afraid that I will be abducted and raped. Hours pass, it becomes late afternoon and I decide to ignore my fears. I hop on my bicycle and bike down my dirt road. I am approaching my last lap of 20. An old man came out, holding his hand up to indicate stopping. The road becomes heavily shaded by the trees. I continue to bike past, feeling sick, waving to him to pretend that he is waving rather than requesting me to stop. He yells to me, "where abouts do you live?" I pretend I can't hear, and continue to bike on.

5 I am racing, my legs pedaling so hard, he's gonna get me, get me, get me. Tears are in full stream down my cheeks. I cut across a neighbors lawn, run to their door, pounding on it. In case he followed I didn't want him to see where I lived. No one's home. God dammit, no one's home. I turn full around, stopping dead. I don't feel my heart, I don't hear anything. My eyes are blurred with tears as I stare across the road at his house, my neighbors house, the

shit brown siding in full view. I see myself standing in his living room, as Beethoven's 9th symphony is being played on me. His fingers running up and down his precious little piano: me. Bum. Bab Buh BUM, he hums as his fingers tickle all over. His favorite keys being the ones over my chest and between my legs.

Oprah is on TV, oh God I wish the characters could see through the TV screen. Oprah help me.

He makes me sit on his lap,

as I can feel he has a hard on. I can look out the window, clutching the worn out of fashion fabric of the sofa with my little fingers of chipped Barbie fashion pink nail polish. I rock back and forth, trying to keep the vomit from coming up. I see my father mowing the lawn, oh God, "Daddy," I whimpered out. My '72 year old, like a grandfather to me' neighbor smiling. "That's right, I'm your daddy, do you like it when I do this? Do you want to see naked pictures of my thirteen year old niece. She has boobies you know, don't you want to see her boobies?" he would ask while his fingers rubbed between my legs, the soft tissue burning. Remembering the way it hurt to pee the next day, sort of like when you got out of a cold swimming pool, and went inside to urinate, how I would hold my breath and let it trickle painfully out of me. Staring down at my little unicorn undies and wanting to throw up again.

I was back on the porch again, the vivid recollections had faded. My fist up in the air in the knocking position. I felt a weight on my chest, my legs felt heavy, my eyesight started to blacken. Down I went on the cold cement porch.

I woke up, dry heaving, my chest blotchy, my mother holding my hand, asking me what happened. I was looking at my legs and arms, bloody, and pink with some thorns from a bush that I ran through apparently scratched me. I hadn't even felt it till now. I lay my head back down, closing my eyes I sighed deeply.

"A dog, a big black dog chased me." I lied.

The TV was on, with a special report about some corrupt catholic girls school, where some nun was fondling the female students. They reported that 70% of pedophiles are ordinary people: teachers, parents, NEIGHBOR'S, baby-sitters, step-parents, siblings, priests, coaches, etc. (Mansfield, 1999). In 1990 there were 119,506 reported cases with a giant leap in 1993 an additional 137,265 cases were reported (Time Almanac 1999); yet 50-90% of all child sexual assaults are never reported. Four million child molesters reside in this country reports the Department of Justice (Ferguson, 1999). Each offender molests an average of 120 victims before their own conviction (Nack, and Yaeger, 1999). Women molest too, as some mothers dedicate themselves far beyond their natural duties of nourishment for children, but will perform cunnilungus on their daughters, fellatio on their sons etc. One in four girls are molested, and one in every five to seven boys are violated as well (Ferguson, 1999). Facts, facts, facts, bombard me. I screamed and ran into my bedroom flushing myself with tears, and sleep.

Place image of "The Scream" by Edvard Munch here

10 I remember reading this book once on survivors of molestation. Some grew up to be excessive drug abusers, alcoholics, prostitutes, suicidal, or even pedophiles themselves. At the end of the book they had anonymous poems submitted for publication. Two poems put me in a fit of rage again.

11 (Polly Flinders)
Little Nettie Glover, snug beneath the covers,
Slept in her cosy little den.
Her father came and woke her, to fumble and to poke her,
12 And make her scared to ever sleep again.

(From *Inside Scars: Incest Recovery as Told by a Survivor and her Therapist*, by Sheila
L. Sisk and Charlotte Foster Hoffman. Copyright 1987, Pandora Press.)

13 This Kind of Touch

Tonight as I lay awake in bed
my hands propped beneath my head,
Afraid to close my eyes in sleep,
for fear that into my room he'll creep.
I see him standing at my door,
as he has so many nights before.
He doesn't think I know he's there;
he doesn't know I see him stare.
And as he moves beside my bed,
his ugly touch I start to dread.
For I feel frightened when I see his hand
reaching out, touching me.
And I think that if I'd never been touched,
it would have been better
Than this kind of touch.

14 I remember sitting in front of the two way mirror, while my neighbors lawyer asked me questions like, "Where did he touch me? Am I sure it wasn't by accident, that his hands didn't just slip? How many times did he touch me?" His red blood shot eyes focused on me, trying to make me look like a liar. I wanted to ask his lawyer if he would trust the man he was defending alone in a room with his own children.

15 One minute goes by, two minutes go by, a child is molested in America every 2 minutes. It's every parent's nightmare, yet it's so many children's reality. Blondie- "One way or another, I'm gonna find you, I'm gonna get you, I'm gonna getcha, getcha,

16 getcha." If he is still alive I know he is coming for me, I know he will drive back in his brown car, to his brown house, to put on his brown boots and look for me. He'll come, sure as shit, he'll come all the way form Connecticut to Vermont, restraining order or no

17 restraining order. He lusts for his little piano. He wants to master his little tune, but all my keys are broken. My stings are out of tune. No more playing I tell you.

18 "Do you like it when I do this? Do you want to see naked pictures of my thirteen year old niece? She has boobies you know. Don't tell your parents that I give you candy, it's our little secret."

19 NEVER eat lemon drops, never ever eat Fig Newton's. Oprah open your eyes, look through the TV, can't you see me Oprah, please, please Oprah see me, see us Oprah. Forget about your book club, and pioneer a kids club. Please Dad, stop mowing the lawn, come to the door dad, Mom call and say dinner is ready, please. Oh God, please don't let him drag me into his room, please, please, God don't let him do it. Oh God, oh please, oh please, oh please.....

OW OW it hurts. Please God, OUCH!

ME

Society is closing in on me. I am shying away from society, developing inside of myself, wanting to die, wanting to kill him, wishing I was never born. I am the lonely child that swings alone on the playground, swaying mindlessly, like a little pendulum; tick tock time goes by collecting its victims. One by one it piles us up in an endless garbage heap like a concentration camp, whispering to us to keep quiet, don't tell what I saw, forget what happened. teach me how to love a man. My parents do it so it must be all right for him to. If I tell no one will believe me anyway, he is a good neighbor, a trusted, respected pillar of the community. I'm just a girl who cries wolf. I'm just a girl deprived of my childhood and sleep. Who do I trust? Not him, he is old, just like my neighbor. Old men like to feel up little girls. So many times when I was little I would wake up screaming or crying covered in sweat. I hated my house it has too many bad memories. This last summer we moved away from it. I never have to see that brown house again except for

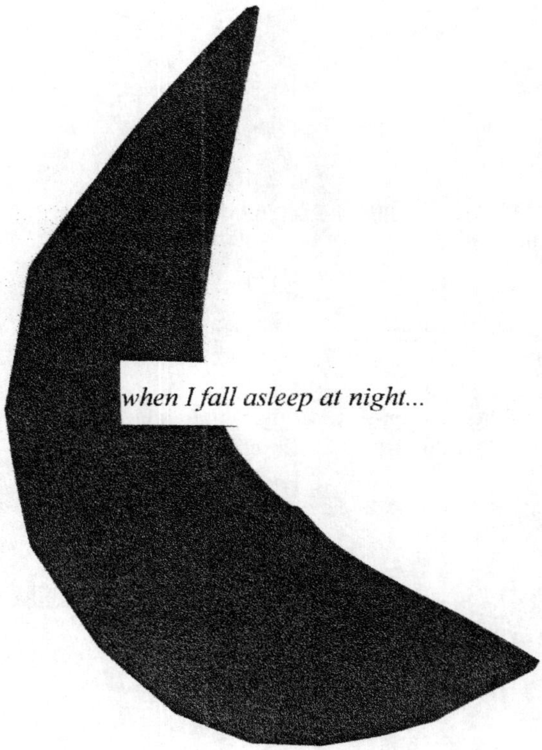
when I fall asleep at night...

Jessica
English 1
March 13, 2000
Bibliography

Crowder, A. (M.S.W) Opening the Door (1993)
Family and Children's Services of the Waterloo Region, Waterloo Ont.
31-33

Elliott, M. Female Sexual Abuse of Children (1993)
The Gulford Press, New York 1, 7, 47

Ferguson, D The Assault on American's Children (1999)
Harbor House (West) Publishers California 1-44

Giannetti C.C. and Margaret Sagarese Parenting 911 (1999)
Broadway Books, NY p. 235

Gordon, S. (Ph.D), and Judith Gordon (M.S.W) Raising a Child in a Sexually Permissive World (2000) Adams Media Corporation, Mass

http://homepages.acenet.co.za/one_small_voice/abuse.htm

http://www.paar.net/sac.html

Lloyd, S. and Liz Hall Surviving Child Sexual Abuse (1993)
The Falmer Press, London 334,335,339

Mansfield, S. "The Avengers On-line" Good Housekeeping
June 1999 vol. 228 No.6 Hearst Magazines p. 122-125, 185

Nack, W. and D. Yaeger Sports Illustrated: "Who's Coaching Your Kid? Every Parents Nightmare" Sept. 13, 1999 vol. 91, No. 10 p. 40-53

Pendergast, W.E. Sexual Abuse of Children and Adolescents (1996)
Continuum, NY p. 26

Time Almanac 1999 (1998)
Borgna Brunner Time Inc. Home Entertainment

Portfolio Narratives

Personal Portfolio Narrative

Rachel Cioffi

To Whom It May Concern:

I am writing to inform you of the portfolio that is in front of you. Included in this portfolio is the work that I have done for the Personal Narrative assignments of Kris Lamoreau's English 001 class. I have put much work into the outcome of these three pieces: "**Once in a Lifetime**", "**A Changing Decision**", and "**Goodbye**". Following is a brief overview of the problems that arose with each piece.

The first assignment was to choose a snapshot that we would like to expand and then expand by adding new details. This paper was to be written in the first person with as much detail as we could remember in the span of one hour of time. My first real problem with "**Once in a Lifetime**" was that I was unsure what to write. I was not able to get across the 'so what' of the story, and I still don't think that I have. My major concern when going to workshop was whether or not the paper flowed. In other words, how were the clarity and the organization. The outcome of the workshop got me nowhere, considering one of the member's thought it was well organized and the other one thought that it needed work. Therefore, I kept the organization as it was and for the revision I changed some grammar errors and added a few details where needed. I think that the final outcome of this paper is still poor, but I was unsure of what to do to get across the 'so what' and why other people would want to read this.

The second personal narrative consisted of a form shift. We were given the option to use the same snapshot or chose a new one. I kept the same snapshot and wrote it in the perspective of my old kindergarten teacher. This piece was entitled "**A Changing Decision**" because what really came out of this story is what I wanted to do as a profession, and that alters the rest of my life. With this piece I did not have as much difficulty as with the first one because I felt that I had an idea of what was wanted. After bringing this piece to workshop, I felt that it was getting old and that there was no way I would be able to use it for the third personal narrative.

The third assignment was to write in the voice of one of our favorite writers. I have always enjoyed the strong voice that Sylvia Plath demonstrates in all of her pieces, especially the poem "**Daddy**". I wrote this final piece about an event that changed my life: the death of my grandmother. I chose this event because I needed to choose something dark because that is Plath's writing perspective. The difficult thing for me to do with this assignment was to actually write the poem. I do not have a very high confidence level for my writing, and writing in this style was definitely a big step. I titled this poem "**Goodbye"** and tried to capture the feelings I had at the funeral. I chose this one to revise for my final personal narrative, which required me changing something about it, so I put it into the third person. The final paper is written as if someone is looking on, and watching this event occur. I had received the suggestion to concentrate more on the rose and tried to do that. After revising this again for the final workshop, I brought it with very low confidence. I felt that it did not flow well at all. My group did not have many suggestions for me on how to change it, although my teacher did. At the end of the second page, my writing was changing from imagery to thoughts, and a poem needs to contain images. So, for the final paper I ended up cutting out a page of the poem and adding a page of prose. In a way, I think that the prose may add to the poem nicely. My major concentration in this piece was to show the emotions of the girl and not to tell them.

I hope that you enjoy this portfolio of my work. I have put effort in trying to create something that has meaning in my life. The two events that I write about in these stories have changed who I am for the better. Thank you for taking the time to read these.

Sincerely,

Rachel Cioffi

WRITTEN expression:

a fairytale story

Tessa Lorenze

Once upon a time there was a young woman at the end of her first year in college. She decided that this particular point in time would be as good as any to declare her major. She marched right up to the Dean of her newfound study and without fear declared, "I wish to change my major to Biological Sciences." She was well received by this Dean and the paperwork was all processed without delay. They then sat down to discuss plans for the following semester's classes. The all-mighty Dean informed this young woman that she would need to take many different requirements. Among this list was a pleasant break from the scientific monotony she would have to endure, it was called English 001, also known as Written Expression.

This young woman brought her list of requirements home to her pleasant one bedroom abode in the Harris/Millis castle (which was rather large, but housing approximately 600 people could be quite cramped at times) and began to create her schedule for the following year. She came to the point when she had to schedule Written Expression and noticed that there were many different sections of this course offered at different times with different professors. The task seemed almost unbearable. "How ever am I supposed to pick the best one?" she wondered. Then a little voice in her head reminded her, "Matty's in this class right now! Go ask him what he thinks!" Without delay she ran over to the South Wing of Harris/Millis, up four flights of stairs and found Matt's suite. She presented Matt with her task at hand and explained the advice she received from the voice in her head and asked if he might be able to assist her in this arduous decision. He said, "My dear Tessa (that is the young woman's name—I forgot to mention that didn't I? Anyway, back to the story) do not stress, your decision is a simple one and you have come to the right place. You see, there is no decision to be made, take the class with Kate Hoffman, she is my professor and I wouldn't recommend it any other way." Quickly she thanked Matty and returned to her wing of the castle without a care in her head.

Now all she had to do was wake up with the sun and punch the numbers into the computer and all would be set for next year.

The night hours went quickly because Tessa had it all figured out and was able to sleep soundly. The morning rolled around and she woke up, turned on the computer, punched in the appropriate numbers and pressed return. Everything was set, or so she thought as she scrolled down the screen, to her surprise she was not allowed into English 001, there was a class restriction. Could it be? Was she too old for this class? The voice in her head once again said, "Go ask Matty." So she did, and he told her to get an override form and show up at the end of his class the next day and just to ask Kate to sign it. He was sure that she would.

The next day rolled around and Tessa walked over to Lafayette from the castle (all the horses were out to pasture so she couldn't round up a carriage) and waited for all of the students to exit the classroom before proceeding. She walked into the room and found a young woman at the front of the class. Tessa thought, my, she looks young, but that must be her. And it was! Kate willingly signed the override and the adventure began.

* * *

Tessa vacationed in Somers, NY for the next three months and quickly found herself back in Burlington, but this time living in a different, but even better, castle. (Her new castle, Christie/Wright/Patterson, was smaller than her previous castle, housing only about 400 people and it even had a "Rotunda" with Pottery Barn couches to lounge on!) She attended her classes and eventually came to English 001 (a.k.a. Written Expression), and found that she was one of the only, if not the only sophomore in the class. But this didn't bother the young woman at all for she had positive feelings about the class from the get-go.

Tessa had set a few goals for Written Expression at the very beginning of the year in a letter to Kate (see Appendix A) among these included just starting to write again. It had been a long time since she had taken an English class, just about two years! Another goal was to receive critical evaluation on her papers, she had recently been writing papers for classes such as Philosophy, on which she had received comments, but only on subject content, not writing quality. Tessa received the exact critical evaluation that she was looking for in this course. She was also excited to experience a different approach to revising and writing papers, which was for sure achieved.

The first task at hand for Tessa was to write a personal essay. She began to get a little nervous because she didn't really think that there were too many significant moments in her life. The little voice in her head wanted to tell her to go ask Matty, but then a different voice reminded her that he transferred to Boston College. However before she could fret anymore Kate had come up with a way to solve this mystery: the Zero Draft. Before she knew it Tessa had come up with a list of many different events that she could focus on.

The personal essay was one of the most enjoyable all year for Tessa. She was able to choose a topic that she knew a lot about and felt comfortable writing about, rock climbing. (For the final product see appendix B) Although at first it was a little difficult to decide whether to focus on her trip to France or her adventures rock climbing in general it was all figured out in time and Tessa was very happy with the outcome. One particular aspect she enjoyed was her description of the Alps the first time she woke up to them. Tessa has never been very adept with details and descriptions but for some reason she has been able to really show and not tell when she wrote about the mountains in France. The following is an example of such a passage.

"I had reached the foothills of the French Alps. I had seen mountains before, but never anything like the ones set before me. They reached so high it seemed as though one could touch the sky from their summit. The landscape began with farms and fields, which led to a backdrop of mountains, who at their base were covered in green trees and terminated in massive slabs of rock at the peak. I had never before been so humbled by nature—Servoz was nothing like I had ever seen in real life, but rather a scene taken from the quaint village in "Beauty and the Beast." The town, as I later learned, was home to only 600 people, but 750 cows."

Another example that we should include in this story of this talent Tessa seemed to have acquired when writing about the French Alps is the postcard description. Tessa struggled and struggled with this assignment because she is usually not sparing when it comes to the use of words. However all of a sudden it just clicked for her and the following became her favorite piece of writing from the whole year (also in Appendix C):

"Looking out onto Aguille-du-Midi the snow seemed like a fresh made bed, something no one should want to disturb. Then quietly a line of ants crept up over the ridge and slowly grew into distinguishable hikers. Although they left fresh tracks behind, the radiating sense of accomplishment justified their disturbance."

Anyway, I think that we have strayed off the topic at hand, back to Tessa's personal essay. Another accomplishment that helped to make this her favorite piece to work on was that she was able to incorporate her present day climbing obsession in Burlington and her first experience climbing in France. This was a difficult balance for her to achieve; however after some serious thought and real revisions it all came together.

Tessa continued to feel positive about her Written Expression class as they started onto their next large assignment, the analytical essay (Appendix D). This was Tessa's least favorite essay, even though she thoroughly enjoyed her topic (the fine music of G. Love and the Special Sauce). She felt as though she set herself up poorly from the beginning with the type of essay she would end up writing and with the task originally set out to accomplish. Tessa sat in Patterson West Wing, trying to figure out what her goal by the end of the paper might be, but she just wasn't so sure.

Then one day in class Kate had her students workshop their essays together. Tessa found this very useful, she workshopped with two other young ladies also in Written Expression, Lulu and Sarah (Appendix E). In this workshop Lulu and Sarah both read Tessa's essays and made some helpful remarks at the end. Tessa realized both when she was reading the essay out loud and also after reading Lulu and Sarah's suggestions that she definitely quoted the songs too often, so she removed a lot of the quotes before her final draft. Another aspect they worked on in this workshop was ridding the essay of weak verbs and adjectives and glossing the essay. All of which helped to make Tessa's final product stronger and more coherent. (However, she still left quite a few weak verbs in her final draft—oops!) Tessa was fairly happy with her final product, she managed to take a different approach to writing her essay and come out with a pretty strong analysis of G. Love's work. Despite this it still was not her favorite essay from the year.

Throughout all of this chaos people call class Tessa had also been occupied by some events in her life, including work, her sister having a baby and looking for a castle of her own for the following year. This last task was kind of on the back of Tessa's mind, but she knew that it would have to come on up to the front soon because her and her castle-mates would have to sign a lease fairly early if they wanted to live somewhere out of the "ghetto." The perfect opportunity came for Tessa when Kate told their Written Expression class they would be spending the next 5 weeks researching a topic of their choice. At first Tessa thought she would have a hard time coming up with a topic for research until the voice in her head reminded her, "You have to search for a castle for next year anyway, why don't you do something that will be of use to you?" So she did.

Tessa had a few difficulties at first with the research part. She went to many different resources (the internet, the Department of Residential Life and the Library, even with all those books) and found them slightly helpful, if at all. But never fear she did not give up. One piece of research that gave her an interesting perspective was the inkshedding she did in class (Appendix F). Not only did Tessa really enjoy answering the questions about other people's topics, but also she liked that she got a chance to read about what each of the other students was researching. Although the inkshedding did not turn out to be as helpful in writing the final product it did help to get a feeling for how the students felt about the housing situation in Burlington. It was interesting to find out that about 75% of Tessa's class stated that they would consider living in on-campus apartments, depending on the rules.

As far as information that Tessa found out that she was able to put in (one of her) final draft(s), she actually even ended up finding out some interesting and new facts. For example, Burlington was rated the number eight city in the country to live in! Who knew, no wonder there are so many people who want to live here! So now that Tessa had finally collected all her data and research she would need she returned to her room in Patterson Castle to write her final draft of the essay. This process for Tessa ended up being a little harder than she had anticipated. Originally her goal was to create this 10-step guide for students looking for off-campus housing (Appendix G). However, once Tessa finished her assignment she did not really feel like she had fulfilled all of the goals that the project intended for her to fulfill, plus she had tons of research that she just couldn't incorporate. So that led Tessa to write a more "magazine type" article (Appendix H). By the end of this project Tessa had been a little frustrated that it took her longer than she expected but she was happy with her result.

Today when Tessa looks back on her fairytale story of Written Expression she knows she has grown as a writer and accomplished her goal of receiving critical evaluations of her work that were helpful. She was also able to target some of her previous "ineptitudes" as a writer, such as description and voice, and come away feeling pretty satisfied with her new found level of achievement. But not only that, perhaps more importantly, Tessa is now an expert on castle hunting in downtown Burlington and will, in no time, be living happily ever after downtown with four good friends.

Final Portfolio

Shawn Delargey

Introduction

For this portfolio I wrote about my semester in English 1. I wanted to write it like an excerption from the course selection book. I know that this book only provides you with a very brief description of the course so instead I pretended that a detailed explanation could be found in the back of the book along with one student's experience in the class and samples of the required work. Hopefully this will be effective. I found it difficult to be very descriptive because I was trying to say what was involved in the class. Although it lacks this, I think that the overall essay is effective and will encourage students to take the course, which was the goal of the article. I think that most people will choose it because your class honestly does improve writing skills and makes writing more enjoyable.

English (ENG)

College of Arts and Sciences

1 Written Expression: A course in writing with some selected readings as examples of style and writing strategies. Three hours. See page 170 for detailed description of course and page 205 for a student's personal experience.

185 English for International Students

5, 6 First Year Semester

001 Written Expression:

This three-credit course, Written expression, focuses on nonfiction writing. The instructor of English one, Kate Hoffman, has many goals for this course. She hopes to introduce writing as a model of learning, along with the process of writing. During the semester, students will develop critical thinking skills and research skills while writing with an awareness of the rhetorical situation. These goals will be accomplished through informal and formal writing assignments throughout the semester.

The informal writing consists of free writes, letters, and journals. Each of these are preformed on a weekly basis. Every class will begin with a free write. During this time, the students will write for a five-minute period without stopping. This exercise aids in getting your ideas down and writing how you *truly* feel about the topic. It is very useful because it does not allow the student time to think what others might want to hear causing them to change their viewpoint. When you write exactly how you feel, your writing is stronger and you really state your case. This will make your views more appealing and/or interesting for the audience. (example found on page 283) This holds true for the letters as well. Almost every week the students will address Kate using a letter format. These letters should also be honest and state how you feel. Although, they must be in a letter format, you have the freedom to write it any style. For example a student can write to the ambiguous "Champ," or state straight facts about her research experience. On pages 284 & 285 , you will find two examples of these letters.

Along with the letters and free write, each student will be required to complete journals for every reading. In these journals the students will be expected to write what they felt added to these essays and what would have made them stronger. This will help the students develop critical reading skills along with improving their writing. By seeing what is and is not effective, they will know what the audience needs in order to be persuaded or interested, and will able to incorporate this into their own writing. On page 286, you will find an example of these journals and on page 291 you will find examples of other in class assignments.

Along with these informal writings, the students will be required to complete a series of formal writing, which are broken down into three main categories. The first is the personal essay. This essay focuses on the use of description and on the writing process. It begins with a biographical incident that you encountered. The next draft you cut that event's time period, so it is only five minutes rather than one complete day. The next major change deals with the narrator. You revise your draft so someone completely different is telling it. All of these drafts will allow you to understand the radical revision process and the importance of details. (example on page 320)

The next portfolio is the interpretive essay in which the students will form an interpretation of a commercial advertisement, movie, etc., and then argue that specific point. It starts with a brief summary of the material and then moves into a close reading of one particular point of your material. (song-verse) Everyone will also write a critical review of the material. This and the interpretations will emphasize critical thinking skills and writing using evidence to support a convincing essay. (example on page 323)

The last formal writing is the research essay. The students will choose a topic and complete both library and field research (interview). After they obtain this information they will write an essay, as it would appear in a magazine. By making the students take advantage of the UVM library's facilities and speaking with a local, the students will familiarize themselves with the resources available to them both here on the campus and in the Burlington area. (example on page 328)

Both the formal and informal writing will aid in the improvement of the students writing skills. Not only will their writing progress, so will their confidence. Writing is a very valuable tool and is used in every profession. When you are confident in what you wrote and how you came about that final product, then your writing reflects that new boldness. I recommend this course to all students, especially first year students. You will learn writing skills in this course, which you will be able to apply to all your other courses. If you still are not convinced on taking this course, you can read about one student's experience in Kate Hoffman's English one class on page 205.

Read one student's personal experience in the following classes:

1 Written Expression:

My Two Feared Words

"Written Expression." I always feared those two words when they appeared separately and now with them together I was petrified. Writing was never a strength of mine and expressing myself was nearly impossible. I mean my opinions about certain topic change daily, so how am I supposed to convince someone how I feel when I am not even sure. Growing up in this fast paced, technological world, how am I suppose to debate with my old school grandfather on specific topics, which we feel completely different about, without him seeing me as the "typical" teenager who speaks without first thinking. It is nearly impossible to verbally do this so how am I supposed to write a paper that will please my "matured," to put it nicely, teacher on how I feel about a particular topic without failing the course? I thought that it could not be done but I learned otherwise in Written Expression.

Why I chose this course, with the title containing my two most feared words, is still a mystery but I can honestly say that I am glad I did. I no longer fear expressing my feelings and attitude on paper. Rather, I find it an exciting challenge to find the exact wording and description that will make my audience curious about my topic and want to continue reading my essays. It is weird that I got all of that from a class I took for a semester but I did.

One reason why I now do not dread writing an essay is because I learned that when you write, you should always be honest. Forget about trying to please the audience, if you do this then your essay will lack strength and credibility. This class also gave me complete freedom on the topic I wrote about. This is also important. If you are writing about a topic that you do not feel strongly about, then your essay will appear dull and lack enthusiasm. This became apparent to me through the informal writing that I did in class. Although I did not love doing all of those assignments I did see how they helped my writing. I saw what worked well in essays and what detracted from the article. I now try to remember this when I am writing. Also getting positive feedback from my peers on what would improve my essay, allowed me to hear what the audience wants and likes in an essay.

I believe that the results and knowledge that I gained from that class appears most distinctively in my formal writing. In this collection of writing, I wrote about personal experiences I had and topics I enjoy. You can see that a little bit of me rubbed off into my writing, even if it was a research paper. Looking back at these three big assignments I see a pattern that I was not aware of before. My three portfolios seem to follow the past, present, future pattern. I did not in any way try this, but it is interesting to see how this course and this semester have changed my life.

In my first portfolio, I wrote about a race I ran in a couple of summers ago (past). I really like this essay because it focused on the use of description. I love painting a vivid picture for the reader, which makes them feel like they were there with me experiencing that moment. Did I write about something that happened in my past because I was nervous about leaving behind everything that was familiar to me and heading to a strange place, which would be my new home? Maybe I was trying to remember my hometown and all of the events, which got me to where I am today.

This race, which is part of my past, was no huge or spectacular event in my lifetime but it is something that I will always remember. If I were to rewrite this draft I would not change my topic. You do not always want to read about this great trip or sad and depressing tragedy. Sometimes you want to read about a situation that occurs daily. One part of this portfolio that I really enjoyed was writing in the "fat business man's" view. I found it humorous and fun to write. Overall I am pleased with my personal essay so lets not dwell on the past but move on to the present.

For my interpretive essay, I wrote about the Jimmy Buffett song, *Changes in Latitude and Changes in Attitude* (present). I am a huge fan of Buffett and listen to his music all the time. It is uplifting and fun. No matter what mood you are in, the instant you hear his voice blaring out tunes, your worries disappear. I would not change my topic if I did this essay over because of this reason. If you really listen to the song, you can see that we should not dwell on the past but live it up in the future. If it is cloudy out, you know that a sunny day is waiting to break through.

Jimmy Buffett's music is part of my life right now. People always say that the music you listen to can tell a lot about a person at that time. Maybe you will sit down and analyze me and make some statement about who I am because I own his CDs. But to me, right now, Jimmy Buffet is something that is familiar to me in this new place. I like to listen to him because he reminds me of home and my background. I am hesitant in my new home and every now and then want something familiar, so I turn on Jimmy Buffett. His familiar lines bring comfort to me and now my future here does not look so dreadful.

In my last portfolio, the research essay, you can see that this hesitation has slipped away and everyday I become more and more accepting and comfortable in my new home (future). In this essay, I wrote about the Burlington Waterfront and how it affects the people in the area. I talked about the people I met down by the lake, the runs I have taken, and sunsets I have seen at the Waterfront. Never did I mention something that I did back home. My paper was centered on Vermont and the people who live here.

This paper made me see all the aspects of the area. Talking with the people, I got to hear real experiences and adventures that took place here along with making new friendships. My research and time by the lake made me realize truly how lucky I am to be living in this beautiful area and that I should take advantage of it. Burlington has so much to offer and this project only brought my attention to this and made me love it up here.

If it took those three portfolios to get me to realize that I really do love it up here, then I would do them over in a heartbeat. Not only have I improved my writing but also I have learned about myself. I now know that I can have a debate with my grandfather or write a paper for my professor and state my opinion in a way which I can grab their attention long enough to show them that I have done my research and am knowledgeable and strongly support this opinion. Hopefully they will recognize that and although they still may not agree with me, they will respect me and my beliefs.

As you can see, my experience in Written Expression has been nothing but positive. Hopefully, after reading this you too will enroll in this course and gain so much from it. My luck to all of you.